THE HEALTH CONSPIRACY

THE HEALTH CONSPIRACY

DR JOE COLLIER

CENTURY
London Sydney Auckland Johannesburg

First published in 1989 by Century Hutchinson Ltd
Brookmount House, 62–65 Chandos Place,
London WC2N 4NW

Century Hutchinson Australia (Pty) Ltd
89–91 Albion Street, Surry Hills,
New South Wales 2010

Century Hutchinson New Zealand Ltd
PO Box 40–086, 32–34 View Road, Glenfield,
Auckland 10, New Zealand

Century Hutchinson South Africa (Pty) Ltd
PO Box 337, Bergvlei, 2012 South Africa

Photoset by Input Typesetting Ltd

Made and printed in Great Britain by
The Guernsey Press Co. Ltd., Guernsey, Channel Islands.

British Library Cataloguing in Publication Data

Collier, Joe
The health conspiracy: how doctors, the drug
industry and the government undermine our
health.
1. England. Drugs. Prescription by general
practitioners
I. Title
362.1'72

ISBN 0–7126–1859–7

To
Rohan
and
James

Always be ready to speak your mind, and a base man will avoid you.

William Blake 1757–1827

Preface

This book is about medicines: how the pharmaceutical industry produces them, how government controls them, how doctors prescribe them and how patients take them. It should be a success story. After all, we now have drug companies well able to develop medicines, a health service devised to provide health for all, a medical profession keen to combat disease, legislation directed towards high standards and politicians who are accountable to the public for their actions. Sadly, however, the book tells a rather different tale, one in which the public is systematically denied its right to see medicines used uncompromisingly in the patients' interest.

My views have been formed over the many years that I have taught about, prescribed, written about and researched on drugs. I have observed the conduct of doctors, politicians and the pharmaceutical industry – and, of course, I have been a patient myself. By revealing the many weaknesses in the system, rather than discussing the strengths, I run the risk of being labelled a pessimist, but I see no alternative way if there is to be change for the better. In order to make any worthwhile advance these weaknesses must be exposed and removed. This book is expressly written to encourage such changes.

A book of this nature has to deal with much more than the problems of the drugs themselves, the story is only complete if the social, political, medical and legal issues surrounding treatment are also covered. By their very nature many of these topics range far outside my own speciality, but to duck them would have made the account incomplete. Rather than leave gaps I have included my 'untutored' views. I hope experts will forgive my forays into their subjects.

However worthy a book's ideals it still has to be written and *The Health Conspiracy* would never have been completed without the boundless support and encouragement of my family, friends and colleagues. My foremost thanks go to my family: Rohan, Daniel, Joshua and Oliver. All have shown great forbearance, never begrudging me those nights and weekends reading, phoning or glued to the word processor. Second I thank Betty Joseph whose painstaking help over many years gave me the wherewithal to tackle and then complete a work such as this.

Many gave advice, granted interviews, lent precious material, shared confidences and helped with source material. They are the pillars of the book without whom little could have been achieved. I am particularly indebted to Aggrey Burke, Frank Delaney, Madeleine Halliday, Andrew Herxheimer, Sue Holland, Martin Jacques, Zarina Kurtz, Beverley Lawrence-Beech, Lea Macdonald, Charles Medawar, Joseph Mirwitch, Patrick Vallance and Andrew Veitch. Others of equal importance must sadly – and for fear of reprisals – go unmentioned. Indeed their need for anonymity constitutes reason enough for writing. I received only one rebuff and the views expressed, none too flattering, also find a place in the text.

Above all I would like to thank James Erlichman, a man of integrity and vision, without whose unstinting and selfless help this book would never have been published. This book is as much his as mine.

INTRODUCTION
The National Stealth Service

As a nation we are hooked on medicines. Each year we blindly swallow millions of pounds worth of vitamins, sleeping tablets, sedatives, cough medicines, antibiotics, tonics and many more. Some of these undoubtedly relieve suffering and save lives; but most have little or no value. Most patients would not know, because they are excluded from their own treatment. Government ministers, not least Mrs Edwina Currie, claim that the public chooses ill health and ignorance – we are a nation of overweights slumped round the telly eating high-cholesterol egg and chips, muddling up our virtually free medicines and forgetting to visit the doctor. When illness strikes, therefore, we have no one to blame but ourselves. Spontaneously we have become a race of medical lemmings.

Or perhaps other forces are at work. Are we suffering instead from a national stealth – a concerted and often clandestine effort by rich and privileged forces who would, out of self-interest, greed or neglect, deny us the treatment, in the widest sense, that we deserve?

From the start, patients find themselves in a hostile environment. They feel ill, their healthy existence is threatened, and they must choose whether to 'bother the doctor'. The visit is filled with further apprehension. It will offer no guarantee of comfort and at the worst it could reveal the truth of a life-threatening illness.

Many patients have told me of their concerns. Commonly they think to themselves: 'The doctor is much too busy to see me. He'll think I'm silly and that I am wasting his time.' But even before this confrontation, the patient has an array of hurdles to face: 'The appointment the receptionist gives me will be just when I have to collect my kids from school. Then I'll be stuck in that tiny waiting room breathing everyone else's germs. When I am finally called, I'll get a doctor I don't know and who will embarrass me.'

And when they get into the consulting room, what chance do patients have to take an active, intelligent and equal part in their own treatment? 'When I speak the doctor seems neither to listen nor understand. He talks down to me, makes me feel inferior, and then expects me to understand some jargon or Latin-sounding names.'

Even so, most patients will tolerate all this. They feel sick and inadequate and doctor, after all, knows best. 'But if I am in such good hands, how come one doctor prescribes pills for my nerves while the other starts by doing blood tests or X-rays?'

How many patients know where doctors get their wisdom from? How many realize that most doctors qualified years ago in medical schools which never required them to consider patients as people. And since then, have been taught much of what they know about new treatment by the paid agents of drug companies who arrive in droves at their surgeries and in the hospitals. Patients may puzzle as to why the doctor's office is festooned with calendars, clocks, paperweights and diaries all stamped with the logos of drug companies. Who has provided the expensive computer in the corner of the room?

'Surely when the doctor needs independent guidance and advice he or she can always turn to the Department of Health?' But for every pound the NHS spends on helping doctors with dispassionate advice, the drug companies spend £50 on propaganda aimed mainly at increasing their sales. And rather than putting real effort behind cervical smears, anti-smoking campaigns and other preventive measures, the government wastes time and taxpayer's money cosseting the drug industry and serving its own political ends.

Patients do care about their own health. But they are being denied access to their own treatment. This book attempts to explain ways in which our health-providers – doctors, drug companies and the government – manipulate the national health to serve their own ends rather than to meet the needs of patients.

CHAPTER 1

Practice Imperfect: The Case Against the Doctors

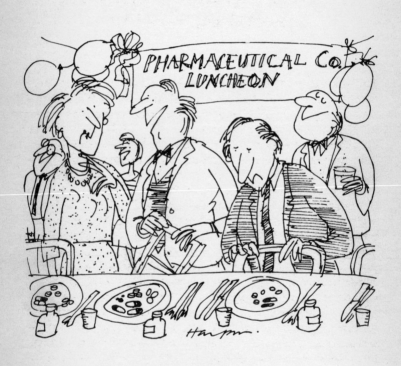

CHAPTER 1

Practice Imperfect: The Case Against the Doctors

Doctors are the pivot of the nation's most important industry: health. They guard their privileges and responsibilities jealously. Patients, fearful, confused and in awe, come to doctors hoping to be made well. Often they fear disability or death, even when their ailment is evidently trifling. Doctors alone hold the magic wand of diagnosis, reassurance and the prospect of a cure.

Governments have traditionally been loath to intrude into this relationship. Only when the gravest allegations are made (as in the Cleveland child sex abuse affair) will the state finally intervene. Normally, the doctor's decisions on diagnosis and drug prescribing are sacrosanct. But doctors wield not just power over their patients' health. They also have substantial control over the public purse-strings, because they dictate which drugs will be bought by the National Health Service – and so which companies will benefit from the £2 billion spent on drugs each year. Pharmaceutical companies, which profit when their products are prescribed, have therefore huge financial motives for seeking to influence doctors in their administration of drugs.

Patients hope that they will get a fair hearing from the doctor, and that diagnosis and treatment will be determined by their needs. What patients do not want is a consultation in which their concerns are ignored or treatment is determined by the vested interests of the medical establishment. As often as not patients' hopes are met. But there are also many occasions when patients remain unhappy, distressingly aware of the gap between how they feel and how the doctor responds. This chapter deals with factors that could be the

3

source of patients' concern. Factors that would influence treatment adversely, and make the patient a pawn, rather than the principal participant, of the relationship.

The Diagnosis

Diagnosis is the first, and arguably most important, step in the therapeutic process. For the patient it brings a sense of order and often reassurance; for the doctor it determines therapy. The process follows a classical pattern. It has three distinct stages; obtaining a history of the complaint, undertaking a physical examination of the patient and finally performing (or having others perform) special tests. Each stage provides diagnostic pointers that need interpretation, and it is in history taking that the scope for interpretation is greatest.

History taking demands a special and personal relationship in which patients express accurately their symptoms without embarrassment or distortion. Good doctors encourage and channel this process without imposing upon it. They are sensitive to the patient's unspoken hints: that hidden agenda of reticence, silences, sighs, or aggression which can reveal more than words. A patient who walks into a surgery with a wound on the hand may simply be patched up by a doctor too harassed or arrogant to probe further. But a sensitive ear might read much into the patient's explanation that 'nothing much caused the wound, the knife slipped while I was doing some handiwork'. This could be a coded plea for help from a severely depressed and suicidal patient. Or, just as tragically, the incident could herald the development of a neurological disease such as multiple sclerosis. Often, the patient's real worry is almost spoken as an afterthought. While getting up to leave the consulting room one patient, whom I was treating for high blood pressure, said 'Oh by the way, over the last few weeks I have started my periods again, I thought I had seen the back of them ten years ago'. Within weeks she was operated on successfully for cancer of the uterus.

The skilled historian can usually elicit and interpret clues with enough expertise to make an accurate diagnosis, but to do this it is important that nothing impedes the flow of communication between patient and doctor. It is therefore

4

poignant that patients' principal complaint about doctors, both in hospitals and general practice, is that they fail to communicate,[1,2] and all too often the doctor is to blame.

Individually, such failures in communication may be difficult to analyse, but overall three reasons dominate, and one of them is the barrier of class.

Class: the prejudice of practice
The political debate has raged, but the truth seems clear. Ill health and poverty go hand in hand. The National Health Service no longer offers, if it ever did, free and equal care to all who need it. Official committees and worthy bodies, in report after report[3,4] have shown that the poor of Britain, in social class five (unskilled manual workers and their spouses), are far more likely to be ill than the rich in class one (professional occupations). The poor are at least twice as likely:

- To suffer gastrointestinal and respiratory symptoms of a chronic nature.*
- To smoke excessively and eat badly.
- To have their children admitted to hospital.
- To have their babies born dead or not survive for more than one week.
- To have, if they are women, cervical cancer or, if they are men, to die of cardiovascular disease.

Even worse, the poor feel powerless to do anything about their chronic disease and increased risk of premature death. To be fair, the poor have faced greater living pain and an earlier grave since the National Health Service began in 1948. But the gap between rich and poor is now getting worse.[5]

Do the poor get worse treatment, in part, because predominantly middle-class doctors fail to treat them sympathetically? It is surely a reasonable question to ask. But even the Black Report, which has proved a seminal publication in the health inequality debate, failed to address this crucial question.[6] Sir

---

Note: Doctors use the terms 'chronic' and 'acute' rather differently from the general public. A chronic condition is one which typically comes on slowly and lasts a long time, for example, rheumatoid arthritis. An acute condition is one which starts and finishes quickly, like a cold. Neither term says anything about the *severity* of the illness.

Douglas Black, for all his skill and wisdom, did not consider whether the poor get sick more often, and suffer longer, because doctors are unable properly to communicate with them and interpret their stories.

Certainly the available evidence shows that doctors are better able to communicate with the rich in social classes one and two.[7] They are more comfortable discussing illness with patients whom they perceive to be intelligent and well-spoken. This is partly because they believe well-off patients will better understand and retain information about the treatment they are given.[8] GPs are more likely to offer well-off patients speedy referrals to specialists, even though the poor might need the expert care even more.[9]

Some working-class people do, however, surmount the social and academic hurdles to become doctors. But they are rare and discriminated against[10], and, moreover, if they are keen to progress they will be advised to change their spots. But to bow to such pressure perpetuates classism in the medical profession and deprives those in social class five of doctors with inherent understanding and the potential to communicate. The class in most need is left without allies.

Medicine must incorporate doctors from all walks of life. Classism is perhaps the most divisive of all medicine's discriminatory practices. Membership of social class five is difficult to define in law, and so legislation equivalent to that on race and gender will not be available to help break down the barriers. Discrimination won't go away unless remedies are sought voluntarily, but there can be little hope while terms like 'a friend of the workers' (once applied to me in an application for promotion), are used to imply criticism rather than praise. So long as doctors remain overridingly middle-class, the plight of patients in the lower social classes looks set to continue.

Sexism: hysteria, the hidden hurdle
Medicine does not limit itself to discrimination against the lower social classes – evidence abounds that it discriminates against women, too. But this is hardly a new problem. The word 'hysterical' comes from the Greek word for 'womb' (ystera) – hence 'hysterectomy'. Hysterical behaviour was

thought to stem from some female disorder of the repro-ductive organs. Women get hysterical. Men get suitably outraged. This myth, discriminating against women, lives on.

It might have been dispelled more quickly if there were more women doctors but the numbers of women in the profession, especially in positions of influence, remains piti-fully and inexcusably low. As many as 80% of all GPs are male, and in hospitals the position is distinctly worse, with men holding 99% of all consultant posts in general surgery and 95% of those in general medicine. The figure is hardly better in specialities where women have a special interest and expertise; 87% of the consultants in obstetrics and gynae-cology are men, as are 79% of those in paediatrics.[11] Had the proportion of women more fairly represented society, then the symptoms and illnesses peculiar to women might not have been left unrecognized, under-researched and under-funded. But the male viewpoint continues to dominate teaching in the wards, in the lecture theatres and in text books,[12] and so attitudes towards women and their concerns remains crude and insensitive.

The picture has begun to change at the undergraduate level, as schools such as the Royal Free and University College London are now admitting women in parity with men. But the improvement has been slow and hampered by opponents. In 1986 almost half (46%) of new medical school entrants in the UK were women,[13] thanks to the Sex Discrimination Act of 1975. But London schools like the Middlesex and the London were still heavily biased toward men,[14] and at St George's Hospital Medical School a computer programme used until 1986 to select students for admission (see page 8) penalised women and made it less likely that they would be selected for interview.[15] In the face of these data, one might imagine that government would set up an enquiry into discrimination against women applying to medical schools. But no, the very idea was dismissed with the line 'there is no evidence in general of discrimination against women'.[16] Hopefully government will rethink its position.

What is more, admission to become a doctor is hardly the whole story. Evidence shows that after qualifying as a doctor the opposition stiffens and the chances of promotion are still severely blighted.[17] Males dominate the promotion procedures, old boy networks ensure men are selected for interview and at interview all the old male devices to put down women continue to be used. Women, for instance, are regularly asked about their personal and private lives (do they plan to have a family, who will look after the children, do they have dependents? etc), and yet no such subjects would ever be asked of their male counterparts. But such questions are the 'privilege' of getting to the interview. Many jobs, at least in university, never get as far as anything so formal. In one London medical school, a third of the professorships over the last six years have been filled without advertisement and with the candidate chosen by word of mouth. Not surprisingly all the 'successful' candidates were men. For the foreseeable future, most doctors in positions of privilege and authority will remain male, and this bias permeates into patient care.

Women patients who come to the surgery with a genuine complaint have to overcome stereotypes. Their illnesses are frequently assumed to be 'all in the mind',[18] while the underlying cause of their genuine illness is ignored. Women are much more likely to be fobbed off with psychotropic tranquillizers than men – for every one prescription for a benzodiazepine tranquillizer written for men, three are written for women.

The problem becomes especially difficult for women who come to their doctors with gynaecological problems, ranging from premenstrual tension (PMT) to the menopause. Premenstrual tension is real. It can cause painful swelling of the breasts, severe headache, uncontrollable irritability and depression so deep that even suicide is contemplated. PMT can also worsen existing diseases such as asthma. Yet most male doctors dismiss this suffering with unqualified derision.[19] Their contempt for post-natal depression is just as great and even more hazardous. Around 10% of women suffer unexplained despair after the birth of even healthy children and need some sort of psychiatric support. To dismiss them is not only cruel, but positively endangers the lives of their newborn children. The infants born to depressed mothers are more likely to suffer not only accidents, but even death.[20]

Even the pain associated with menstruation remains almost

totally under-researched. This is hardly surprising, perhaps, when all of the leading gynaecological textbooks in Britain are written by men. Imagine, if you can, what resources of money and brain power would be thrown into a medical condition if, once a month, men were debilitated by deep throbbing pain and bleeding from their sexual organs. No expense would be spared to save them from this disabling condition!

Childbirth is fraught with the same lack of communication between doctors and mothers-to-be.[21] It is not simply that pregnant women think that they know what is best for themselves and their babies. When a normal function such as childbirth has become enveloped in drip sets, catheters, monitors and electrodes, introduced into the most personal of places, it seems hardly surprising that there has been a plea from women for a more 'natural' childbirth.

The medical establishment has looked upon this genuine complaint with suspicion. It wants nothing to do with women who, in growing numbers, arrive on labour wards with a familiar shopping list of demands, telling doctors and midwives what to do. The women want a natural childbirth. What on earth, they ask, does this mean? This year it is having the baby in the squatting position. Last year it was underwater and the year before it was labour in the dark. 'Next year,' said one consultant paediatrician, 'it should be hanging from the chandeliers.'[22]

Sexual prejudice even determines research policy. The Medical Research Council, which has nurtured many Nobel Prize winners, recently mounted a major study on the treatment of high blood pressure. Part of its enquiry concentrated on the unwanted effects of the drugs used, and amongst the topics raised was the effect of treatment on patients' sexual function. This was a perfectly sensible approach, since people taking drugs for high blood pressure typically stay on them for life and any permanent loss of libido could be extremely distressing. More than 200 doctors contributed to the study, which cost £4.5 million to mount and involved 17,354 patients. For most of the unwanted side effects of these drugs, men and women were considered equally. But when it came to measuring the loss of sexual desire, no one thought it to ask the women patients how they felt. The study that a significant number of males taking the heart ㅁ propranolol, became impotent. The figure was similar for those males taking a diuretic called bendrofluazide. In all probability, women in the study will also have been affected. But no one in the male-dominated medical world bothered to ask them.

Racism: the black and white barrier

The third major barrier to communication between doctors and their patients is racial prejudice. Racism abounds in British society and it is no less prevalent among doctors. It is deeply rooted in the structure of the medical profession, beginning in our medical schools when students are selected and then continuing through to consultant appointments and the allocation of extra payments for the most senior members of the profession.

Ethnic minority groups have long complained about a racial bias in the selection of medical students. It took a survey on the composition of students at the London medical schools to confirm their suspicions.[14] The study published in 1986 showed that the proportion selected from ethnic minorities varied widely between the medical schools but that in any one school the racial pattern was consistent. At the Royal Free Hospital Medical School in London, 17% of the students in 1986 were from ethnic minorities (the figure for doctors practising in the UK as a whole is 25%). At the Westminster Hospital Medical School the picture was quite different – only 5% of its students were non-white. Such raw statistics, however alarming, were only an indicator until the discovery at St George's Hospital Medical School that a computer program used to select applicants for interview had been deliberately weighted against students from ethnic minorities. This was particularly disturbing because, in the earlier survey, St George's was shown to be one of the more liberal schools, with an ethnic minority proportion second only to that of the Royal Free.

Information from the application form, such as the student's name, ethnic origin (based mainly on the name), age, gender, exam results, hobbies, handwriting and the head teacher's report, was fed into the computer which then derived a score for the particular applicant[15]. The lower the score, the better the applicant was judged to be. Anybody with more than forty points, roughly speaking, was not asked to come for an interview, and so automatically failed to get through the first and most critical hurdle in the admissions process. Unbelievably, the computer was programmed to add to the student's final score up to 17 'penalty' points for anyone of 'non-caucasian' origin. So, if applications were processed for two students who were identical in all respects apart from their names, then if the one called Smith scored 25, the one called Patel would be given a score of 42. Smith alone would be called for interview.

Several important lessons about institutionalized racism were learnt from this incident and from the inquiry that followed[15], and such lessons have implications way beyond the medical profession. First, in any establishment it only takes two or three members of staff with roles central to an admissions procedure to run a clandestine policy of discrimination. Second, where such a hidden element has been created, it will only be broken by those alive to discriminatory practice. St George's had indeed made attempts to ensure student selection was fair by setting up two working parties to examine admissions policy. But what did the two working parties have in common? All the members of the working parties were white and male.

The Commission for Racial Equality estimated that the discriminatory programme will have reduced the number of successful non-white applicants to St George's by up to 30% each year. And remember, St George's is a relatively enlightened medical school. We do not know what mechanisms might have been used at other schools, but when St Mary's Hospital Medical School was asked why non-whites had only one-third the chance of a white applicant of being called for interview, the school replied that they were turned down because of their 'non-academic suitability'.[23]

Following the St George's inquiry, Lord Flowers, Vice-Chancellor of London University, decided to probe into the admissions procedures at all colleges.[24] This step, plus the decision by the Department of Education and Science to include a question on the student's ethnic origin in the university (UCCA) application form[25] should make discrimination less likely.

Racism does not stop at medical school. Once qualified, ethnic minority doctors then find jobs more difficult to come by both in hospitals[26] and in general practice.[27] Attitudes that I have heard, such as 'He is Indian, but he is very clever' when describing a colleague, or 'Oh, not another Patel' when shortlisting candidates for a job, are commonplace, even among those who see themselves as liberal and egalitarian. And in such an environment it can be no surprise that even when non-whites *do* succeed against the odds, they tend to be directed to what doctors see as the 'less popular' specialities like geriatrics and radiology,[28] because in these specialities ethnic minority doctors are over-represented. Even when they reach consultant level, when professional equality should have become established, doctors from the ethnic minorities are less likely to get extra salary (merit) awards, and less likely to sit on any of the policy-making committees.

Racism within the profession does not necessarily mean that doctors will have racist values when they come to treating patients. But the chances are high and in reality it would seem inevitable.[29] This is doubly important because some physical diseases are distributed differently amongst the races. Immigrants from the Caribbean have a particularly high mortality from tuberculosis, liver cancer, high blood pressure, stroke and diabetes. Responses to drugs may vary from race to race. Eskimos and the Japanese are particularly good at breaking down certain medicines, such as the drug to reduce high blood pressure, hydralazine, while the Mediterranean Jews have a rather poorer capacity. In addition, some illness may be the result of particular customs: Hindu Asian women living in the UK are particularly likely to develop vitamin D deficiency during pregnancy if they adhere strictly to their traditional diets.[30]

It is hard to say exactly how much racism unfairly affects patient care, but a Health Education Council report found that 'racial discrimination (in the NHS) reduces access to services, causes unnecessary suffering, discomfort and probably deaths'.[29] The report implicates doctors in this process by suggesting that, when dealing with ethnic minority patients, doctors 'make racist comments in earshot of the patient . . . address patients in a derogatory manner', offer 'poor or no explanations', often assume that the patients 'are faking or hypochondriacs' and perform an 'inadequate or no examination before diagnosis and prescription of treatment'.

A lamentable lack of awareness of ethnic minority issues is revealed in a series of articles in the *British Medical Journal*. The series, while looking at many aspects of the diagnosis and management of illness, found it necessary to remind doctors working with patients from ethnic minorities that they '. . . should avoid stereotyping and appreciate that each individual's responses and adaptations to Britain are unique',[31] that they should avoid mispronouncing or mis-spelling names because this is 'annoying' and causes 'a loss in personal dignity'; that 'staff must be sensitive to the various problems which may arise in relation to diet, clothes, the wearing of jewellery or objects of religious significance'.[32] Such caveats could only have meaning in a society that is racially intolerant and poorly integrated.

Even when doctors know that they are studying diseases and conditions which are crucially affected by a patient's race or religion, they demonstrate woeful ignorance. One survey showed that only four of 25 articles and letters published in the *British Medical Journal* correctly defined the racial, religious and cultural backgrounds of the 'non-white' patients involved.[33] Africans, West Indians, Bangladeshis and Pakistanis were all lumped together as one. This is not merely tactless. It is medically inept.

The clearest evidence of medical racism is found in psychiatric illness, where appreciation of the patient's mood and history alone determine diagnosis. Black people in Britain who visit their GPs with evident emotional problems are less likely to be given a referral to a psychiatrist.[34] Presumably they are more often judged to be feckless, faking it, or spaced out on marijuana and would, therefore, be wasting the psychiatrist's valuable time. Yet if admitted to hospital, people of Afro-Caribbean origin are more likely to be diagnosed as schizophrenic, more likely to be given electroconvulsive therapy and more likely to be given high doses of medication.[35] They are also more likely to be 'sectioned', that is to say compulsorily detained in a mental hospital against their will under the Mental Health Act 1959[36], and, if sectioned, more likely than whites and other racial groups to get put into a special security unit where they are virtually imprisoned under lock and key.[37]

Classism, sexism and racism are probably the three main bars to communication and so to the provision of the best medical advice. There are, of course, others, such as religion and homosexuality, and with the sectarian problems in Northern Ireland and the AIDS epidemic centred on the major cities, these too need to be faced with growing urgency.

Disease and drugs: the blinkers of conventional medicine
Doctors also fail patients because they are preoccupied with, even obsessed by, disease. Right from their earliest days at medical school, training concentrates on the recognition and treatment of disease, rather than its prevention. It is common to hear of patients who come to the clinic with symptoms that seem trivial being treated as an irritating waste of time. Healthy people who merely want to learn how to prevent illness are treated even more harshly – unless the doctor can claim an extra fee for the rare forms of preventative medicine which are permitted under the NHS. GPs get paid £6.90 for cervical smears taken in women of a set age and at set intervals. But no such fee is offered outside the defined programme, and so a woman who just wants a check-up to put her mind at rest, or to spot the early symptoms of a cancer, may get short shrift. This approach is the same for all illness, except that in the young where for years there has been a programme to check the development of all children up to the age of 16. In the main the only legitimate way that a 'healthy' adult can obtain a check-up is as part of an examination for an insurance policy, but this too is considered an extra, and the patient will be charged.

Disease is so much a part of a doctor's horizon that it may be difficult for a patient to escape the consulting room without an illness being diagnosed and at least one medicine being prescribed.[38] In fact, it is hard to escape the conclusion that some doctors almost feel obliged to invent illness. For example, a quarter of all the women in one inner London area were recently being treated for psychiatric disease![39] Living in poorer areas where unemployment, bad housing, domestic violence and broken homes are common puts women who are trying to keep their families together under considerable stress. But a widespread diagnosis of mental illness is clearly ridiculous. Yet this is not an isolated example. Another study revealed that more than half the elderly patients admitted to the medical (not psychiatric) wards of one Newcastle hospital had been prescribed tranquillizers (benzodiazepines) by their GPs.[40] Even healthy women get the blanket drug treatment. Most pregnant women who come to hospital to have their babies are given some form of sedation on the night before delivery. One has to ask: who are the drugs really for – the mother-to-be, her baby, or the medical staff who want a quiet night?

Of course there are also good reasons too why doctors are trained to focus on disease. The whole art and science of history-taking is designed to discovery quickly whether anything is 'wrong' with a patient. This is the critical phase because if, after hearing the history and conducting an examination, nothing is discovered, then a patient may be sent away with a few words of reassurance. But it is harder than you might think for a doctor to tell a patient that nothing is wrong. There are several reasons for this. First, most patients prefer a diagnosis that tells them what ails them. They want something firm to grasp, unless the truth is worse than their fears. And they want to leave the surgery with a medical wonder cure that will painlessly erase their doubts and cure their symptoms.

Doctors too need to find reassurance in their own diagnoses. If they simply dismiss a patient as healthy they must live with the nagging fear that they have missed something. If they can define an illness, they can share it with the patient who may then, in diseases like diabetes or asthma, become responsible for the daily administration of their own treatment. A firm diagnosis also gives the doctor intellectual satisfaction. Faced with a puzzle, the doctor wants to solve it. Patients seldom see this side of things. These little, daily triumphs keep doctors sane and keep them going.

The treatment that patients receive can then, however, be frighteningly arbitrary. In a few illnesses, like leukaemia and tumours of the lymphatic system, treatment is virtually dictated by a national, standard therapy. But for most illnesses it is determined only by the particular views and even prejudices of the individual doctor. Take, for example, the common illness, tonsillitis. Figures show that some surgeons seem to do little else but remove tonsils and adenoids,[41] while others believe the operation is either useless or positively harmful and virtually never perform it. Part of the reason for this is that with few exceptions no serious attempt has been made to define standards of treatment across the NHS. Until patients, as consumers, demand a review of clinical practice, discrepancies in treatment will go unchecked. It will be impossible to tell if doctors who prescribe unusual therapies do so because they are therapeutic leaders or laggards.

We do have one clue about whether doctors have become insensitive robots cut off from their patients, and ironically it has come from that impersonal instrument, the computer. Patients with severe abdominal pain were asked to 'diagnose themselves' by answering step-by-step questions put to them by a computer. The conclusions made by the computer as to whether surgery was necessary, proved more reliable than conventional diagnoses made by their own physicians.[42]

Medical training must begin again to stress more strongly those aspects of therapy that depend so much on communication, sharing and empathy. In my view the General Medical Council (GMC), the body responsible for medical education, has failed us. The medical profession is poorly equipped to communicate with the most ill groups in society (social class five), and when faced with the articulate patient who demands details of treatment options it ducks and weaves and tries to withdraw. The British Medical Association has a policy, for instance, of *not* producing detailed guidelines on specific treatments. It recognizes that guidelines would help doctors but is frightened lest they get into the hands of patients. A questioning informed patient is the last thing doctors want.

Of course the GMC surveys what is happening in the medical schools[43] and produces broad recommendations[44] on what students should be taught and how they should relate

to patients and colleagues, but in so many re
urgency and offers no clear leadership. The mes
ivory tower seems to be 'leave medical educati
assume that public demands will go away'. B
changing. Medical schools must recognize the ~~sponsi-
bilities to society. Selection procedures and teaching must
address the problems of classism, sexism and racism. Doctors
must recognize that the public has rights, and that patients,
although ill, must maintain their autonomy.

Read with envy the advice given by the New Zealand authorities to their medical schools:[45]

- Doctors must recognize that they are socially account-
able to their community.
- Therapy should be patient-centred, with patients
treated as equals.
- Doctors should understand that in a multicultural
society, education dominated by the values of one
culture will fail to address multicultural health
problems.
- Doctors must learn to take into account women's
perspectives on health.

Drug Dependence: Doctors' Addiction to a Chemical Cure

Once the history has been taken and the diagnosis made, the
next step is treatment, which for the most part will be drugs
– sometimes known as the 'doctor's friend'. The easiest way
to keep patients at arm's length is to write them out a quick
prescription and send them on their way. We all know the
stereotype of the lazy GP. He can barely bother to look up
when you come in. He fiddles with his pen while you explain
your problems. He cuts you short, mutters something incom-
prehensible, scribbles illegibly on his pad and ushers you from
the surgery with the advice: 'Get these from the chemist and
come back in a week if you don't feel any better.' Only when
you get to the chemist and ask the pharmacist do you find
out what is wrong with you and what the pills are supposed
to do.

Do doctors know all that is necessary when they select the
best drug to prescribe? Sadly, the answer is no. Even the

most conscientious and caring doctor cannot possibly have a good working knowledge of all the 4,000 prescription drugs listed in the *British National Formulary* – the handbook provided free and published jointly by the British Medical Association and the Pharmaceutical Society.

Why are there so many drugs on the market? Because the pharmaceutical companies are constantly pouring out new products. Are they all wonder cures, or even useful drugs better than their predecessors? The answer, firmly, is no. Take, for example, the treatment of anaemia, a common condition. For the vast majority of patients effective treatment can be given with either iron, folic acid or vitamin B_{12}. All we really need is four or five different formulations of each of these medicines for administration by injection or mouth to adults and children. Yet the doctor is faced with more than 100 different preparations of these basic drugs made as mixed preparations or as single agents. How can doctors possibly choose? Again, the answer is that they cannot. Most GPs, in fact, restrict themselves to prescribing, across the whole range of illnesses, no more than 200 or 300 different drugs with which they feel familiar.

The drug companies battle with each other to get doctors to switch to their own brands. The fight for market share is fierce, expensive and not always ethical. In the next chapter, we shall see how one of the world's largest drug companies, Bayer of West Germany, was caught bribing British doctors to switch to its own brand of heart drug. Even without under-the-table inducements, the drug companies collectively spend an estimated £5,000 a year on each GP to promote their branded medicines.

But to make a rational selection between any two medicines a doctor does not want advertising hype. He or she needs detailed and dispassionate information that will compare the drug's safety, efficacy (how well they actually work), convenience to take, uniformity of quality and also their comparative cost.

You might reasonably expect that the Department of Health would be the independent arbiter ready and willing to give this essential advice. But until now, little direct help has come from government. This may seem astonishing. The doctor, plagued by drug salesmen, cannot turn to the NHS for advice on which drugs are likely to be best for the patient. At the Department of Health there is a body called the Committee on the Safety of Medicines, or CSM for short. Keep it in mind, because it is at the heart of this book and the way prescription drugs are controlled in Britain. (In the United States, similar regulatory work is done by the US Food and Drug Administration). The CSM is obliged, before new drugs are marketed, to assess their safety compared to other equivalent products. It is also obliged to establish a drug's quality and when it is a 'generic' to guarantee that a new formulation provides an identical amount to that delivered from the original brand leader. But, astonishingly, the CSM has no responsibility under the Medicines Act to consider 'relative efficacy'. In other words, it has no right to say whether a new heart drug for high blood pressure is as good as those already on the market, and, even if it isn't, it will almost certainly still allow the drug to be prescribed. Nor can the CSM make any judgments about a new drug's cost or its convenience in use. So, if a new drug is 'safe' – that is to say, if the harm it might do is 'acceptable' – and its batch quality is consistent, then it can still end up on the market even if it is absurdly expensive, difficult to swallow and does not work as well as cheaper and more palatable drugs.

Without help from the government when selecting drugs, what is a caring, but often confused, doctor supposed to do? There are a few publications which help. Both the *British National Formulary* and the *Drug and Therapeutics Bulletin* (published by the Consumers' Association) do give dispassionate advice. Most hospitals also have their own drug and therapeutics committee which advises on the latest medicines. But for GPs, who prescribe 80% of drugs given to patients, such advice is either not available or buried under the welter of advertising and promotional material with which the drug companies bombard every surgery in the land. In general, there can be few physicians with the time, interest, expertise or resources to fully acquaint themselves with the necessary information when choosing between one drug and another.

The limited list

Help has now arrived – in a limited way, and from motives that may have little to do with patients' wellbeing. In April 1985 the government introduced a so-called limited list of drugs that would henceforth be prescribed under the National Health Service.[46] The limited list covers only seven out of the several hundred therapeutic areas of medicine (cough and cold remedies, antacids, pain killers, vitamins, laxatives and apperiants, bitters and tonics, and the sleeping tablets and sedatives belonging to a group of drugs known as the benzodiazepines). Many critics believe that the list was introduced only as a cost saving exercise, and saw the step as driving a wedge between the rich, who would buy their own expensive drugs and the poor, who would be stuck with inferior medicines from the list. The very idea of the National Health Service appeared to be under threat.

Whatever the original intention, the list finally chosen included those drugs in each category that were the best in terms of safety, efficacy and cost. In these categories at least, therefore, it merely requires doctors to prescribe those drugs available on the NHS. To go outside the list risks using a product that might be ineffective or possibly even dangerous.

The pharmaceutical industry, as one might expect, fought vigorously to stop the limited list from being implemented. It mounted an expensive advertising campaign in the press and sent legions of lobbyists into Whitehall and Parliament in a vain attempt to thwart the government's plan. The industry gave every impression of being concerned about the nation's health. But more cynical observers thought its real fear was that its profits would suffer if many of its unnecessary and expensive products were banned from the NHS prescription pad. The government claims to have saved around £75 million each year on the NHS drugs bill.

Just as importantly, doctors can, for the first time, prescribe without confusion, knowing that their patients are getting only the best drugs available. Many doctors, however, backed by the British Medical Association, opposed the list; they feared it restricted their freedom of choice. This notion is emotive rather than real, because freedom of choice is not real, since, as we have seen, such freedom requires that the doctor has the appropriate knowledge, and knowledge depends on access to information and the time and skill to decipher it.

Inevitably doctors must rely on the judgement of others. The limited list ought now to be extended to cover all the therapeutic groups of medicines. So far, the government has shown no political will to do so. In the meantime, some health authorities have drawn up their own lists and encourage doctors to stick to them. In Wandsworth, where I work, we set up our own list long before the government acted[47] and as a result we will almost certainly have saved lives. Five of the six anti-arthritis drugs which were eventually withdrawn by the government on safety grounds (feprazone, Osmosin, zimeldine, zomepirac and nomifensine) were never made freely available for prescription in our hospitals. Furthermore we have saved an estimated £1.1 million between 1981 and 1988 on our drugs bill – a very useful sum at a time when the National Health Service is being starved of resources.

Alternative medicine: complement or curse?
If most doctors find it hard to choose between conventional drugs, they become even more confused when facing the claims made for the bewildering array of alternative therapies ranging from acupuncture and reflexology to homeopathy and herbal cures.

Just as there are around 4,000 branded conventional medicines available in Britain, there are an additional 4,000 or so herbal and traditional medicines to choose from.

Doctors trained in orthodox medicine are taught to distrust so-called 'quacks' and their weird remedies. Some of this mistrust is well-founded. Some is not and is merely a disguised form of 'restrictive practice'; doctors, like all skilled workers, are suspicious of iconoclasts who challenge their status as the people's only proven healers. Let us try to distinguish between prejudice and understandable caution.

Conventional medicine is the best form of treatment for many diseases. Antibiotics, although often misused, are a genuine wonder cure for life-threatening infections. It is positively criminal to withhold them from a patient suffering, for instance, from tuberculosis, diphtheria, or bacterial meningitis. It would be irresponsible to allow a person with infections such as these to infect others just because he or she did not believe in antibiotics and preferred to seek alternative treatment. In the same way, it is wrong to impose alternative medicine on an epileptic child when conventional medicines like phenytoin, carbamazepine or sodium valproate are so effective in controlling this frightening and dangerous condition.

However, there are still many diseases, for example rheumatoid arthritis, sciatica, and the various allergies, against which conventional medicines often provide inadequate relief, and may even cause unwanted effects so severe as to be worse than the original complaint.

Psychosomatic illnesses have proven just as difficult to treat with conventional drugs. Doctors are rightly criticised for their gross overuse for many years of the hypnotics and sedatives such as Valium and Librium. Rather than attempting to attack the root cause of a patient's symptoms, too many times doctors have prescribed these best of best friends to get the patient out of the clinic or alternatively to help patients paper over the cracks in their lives.

Why have they done this? Some doctors are lazy and incapable of dealing with their patients as people. Others feel swamped by surgeries full of people who, in generations past, might have turned to their families or other 'carers' in the community for support rather than to tranquillizers.

When conventional treatment does not work, many doctors feel they have failed. Inevitably, they may ease their own anguish by reducing the time they spend with patients they cannot help. Instead of care, they offer only repeat prescriptions. The vicious circle begins. Patients who feel neglected may turn increasingly to alternative forms of medicine where at least they receive more time from 'the healers'. A common feature of many of the complementary approaches is that they claim to be natural and involve a rather close physical or emotional 'caring' relationship between the patient and the therapist. There is often touching, and there is always time – not least because, it must be accepted, the patient is paying for the attention he or she receives.

The importance of caring alone in helping to cure people

of illness cannot be overestimated, either in conventional or alternative medicine. Carefully controlled trials using conventional procedures have consistently revealed how the very act of caring significantly affects disease processes. For example, placebos (substances which are inert and have no known pharmacological value) will heal 40% of peptic ulcers or prevent exercise-induced asthma. Yet if the placebo is withdrawn patients may suffer withdrawal symptoms. The mind is a powerful healer. Placebos can even significantly reduce the chest pain of heart disease.

Indeed, it has even been demonstrated that placebos can cause unwanted side-effects. Reports of impotence, lethargy, weakness, headache, nausea and rashes in patients taking placebos are common. It is even accepted by many orthodox doctors that the timing of the onset of many of the most threatening diseases (cancer, heart disease and so on) can be related to severe psychological upset, such as the death of a close relative, divorce, unemployment or even moving home. So it may well be that stress-related diseases can be allayed by the close relationship which so often develops in the alternative or complementary approach to medicine.

Besides, many 'alternative' medicines do have a real effect on the body's function and over time have been incorporated into conventional treatment. Acupuncture, for example, appears to increase the levels of enkephalins, the body's own morphine-like substance, which relieve pain and alter the mental state. Osteopathy has much in common with physiotherapy and sports medicine. While recently homeopathic (disappearing) concentrations of antibodies have been reported to have a real effect on the body's immune system.[48] But even the most liberal of conventional doctors may find it hard to discover evidence for any real healing effect from magnetism, radionics, and reflexology – all alternative therapies which command allegiance among some satisfied customers. But then conventional medicine also finds it hard to explain the benefits provided by psychoanalysis and other forms of psychological treatment such as behavioural therapy.

If conventional medicine often fails, and alternative medicine is, at worst, harmless, why is it scorned by the medical establishment? We have seen that prejudice plays its part. But we have also seen that alternative medicine can be dangerous if it deprives seriously ill people of life-saving drugs such as antibiotics. Moreover, herbal medicines are not always harmless. Many of them, just like conventional drugs, have unwanted side effects. Some of these are relatively trivial. Juniper can cause diarrhoea, and camomile and yarrow can produce rashes, but broom, for example, may induce abortion, comfrey and coltsfoot have been linked with inducing cancer,[49] and the Indian herb, linn is associated with catastrophic blood loss.[50] Incorrect manipulation by alternative therapists has damaged joints and acupuncture can cause severe internal bleeding and carries with it the risk of disease transmission from infected needles.

The real problem is that we just do not know enough about 'fringe' remedies because most have never been subjected to the same rigorous testing which we expect before a conventional drug is permitted on the market. The manufactures of herbal medicines say they do not have the huge resources of the pharmaceutical industry and they simply cannot afford to subject their products to the same tests for safety and efficacy. The problem has come to a head because the government at first seemed to order that all medicines (conventional and herbal) would have to pass similar product licence review (PLR) by 1990. But the herbalists were able to command impressive support in the House of Commons and the rules have now been changed. On advice from the Medicines Commission and the Committee on the Review of Medicines, the Department of Health ruled that herbal and traditional medicines used for minor, self-limiting disease would have to pass the tests for quality and safety applied to conventional drugs. But crucially, they would not have to pass the limited laboratory tests for efficacy used to show that conventional medicines work. Instead their makers would normally only have to point to 'pharmacological rationale and bibliographic evidence'.[51] These are fancy words for what amounts to relying on tradition and hearsay.

Allowing herbal treatments to escape tough scientific scrutiny is just is not good enough. There are unscrupulous herbalists just as there are unsavoury medical practitioners. Some herbal products do contain concealed contaminants. Others do not even contain the herbs listed on the label. Besides we simply need to know how, and if, herbal remedies work. No government can shirk from this duty and a complete review of herbal medicines and all other forms of complementary medicine is well overdue. A recent survey in *Which? Magazine* (produced by the Consumers' Association), reported that vast numbers of people at some time in their lives turn to complementary medicine[52] because they feel that conventional doctors and conventional drugs have failed them.

Medicine is now facing a crisis of confidence. Doctors have lost their touch and in the consulting room can no longer make diagnoses with confidence. Rather than turn to preventive medicine or supportive therapy, services which they are particularly well placed to offer, GPs have been seduced into prescribing increasing numbers of medicines whose risks and benefits they don't fully understand. Patients seem to have recognized the dilemma and are turning to 'alternative' medicines in which practitioners appear to know what they are doing, where there is no obvious intellectual or emotional barrier between practitioners and patients, and where the patient sees little risk of harm.

In the next chapter we examine how the drug companies, which I believe have helped draw doctors away from patients, have come to exert their unwholesome influence over our national health.

CHAPTER 2

In the Pocket of the Industry

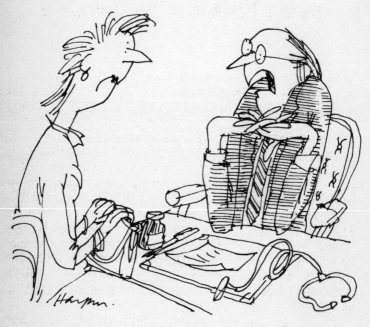

Look at it this way Mrs. Gibson – if you keep taking the pills I'll feel so much better

CHAPTER 2

In the Pocket of the Industry

The single most dominant influence on medical practice is now the pharmaceutical industry. It provides not only the medicines needed for improving and maintaining health but its influence insinuates itself in the fabric of medical research, post-graduate education and medical practice itself.

The prize for the industry is the £2.1 billion which the National Health Service will spend on medicines in 1988 – one tenth of its entire budget. General practitioners are the principal target of the drug industry's attentions, because they write 80% of all prescriptions. Half of the money which the Department of Health spends on general practice goes straight into the hands of the drug companies. Hospital doctors may spend less on drugs because they see fewer total patients, but they are often the opinion formers who will influence which drugs GPs prescribe, and so they are courted just as assiduously.

To win this business, pharmaceutical manufacturers now spend £180 million a year on drug promotion to doctors. In addition, they donate large but unspecified amounts towards the research and other costs of both universities and the health service. The great influence which the drug companies exert to get their products prescribed over rival brands has been revealed by various studies of doctors' prescribing habits.[1] Advertising agencies also like to boast that their campaigns boost the sales revenue of their clients. There was no control over this excessive promotion until the Medicines Act of 1968 was passed in the wake of the thalidomide scandal. But the law's weaknesses and loopholes are still being exploited.

Since drug companies exist to make money and to do this they must sell medicines, the pharmaceutical industry adopts a very different attitude towards illness from that of patients or the medical profession. Patients want health, doctors want cures, drug companies want profits.

In general practice, medicines are the mainstay of treatment. In hospital practice, though vitally important, they compete with alternative forms of treatment such as surgery and psychotherapy. In either setting the decision on whether and what to prescribe depends on four standard factors: the patient, the doctor, the pharmaceutical industry and the government. Of these, industry dominates the decision-making process. It alone has a clear and unambiguous goal: to manufacture drugs and promote and perpetuate their use so as to generate profit. In general the attitude of doctors and government towards the use of medicines is dithering and divided, and over the years they have offered little effective opposition to the resourceful, efficient and often ruthless machine that works to keep the industry profitable.

The need to make money, rather than a primary desire to cure disease, drives and directs drug development. To guarantee their continued prosperity, drug companies, like other businesses, have to provide their customers with attractive lines. Profit motives determine the industry's policies on research, manufacture and marketing. If any particular project is not producing adequate returns it is likely to be axed. In planning the research programme, predictions are made as to which areas of development are likely to lead to greatest profit. Initial calculations consider the prevalence, duration and global distribution of the target illness. Later equations focus upon marketing and promotion. The company will determine the drug's image and attempt to establish a unique selling point on which to base its promotional campaign. Then, taking into account the perceived need for the drug and whether similar drugs are also available from competitors, the company will determine a price that the consumer will bear, whether it be an individual private patient in the United States or a monopoly buyer such as the National Health Service in Britain.

Drug companies are most frequently attracted by projects that will lead to, for example, the development of a medicine for the life-long treatment of a common chronic condition (for example a new aspirin-like drug for arthritis). Contrariwise a medicine that could only be used for a rare condition of short duration occurring in the elderly would not be favoured.

In addition to a wide application, a new drug would ideally also have a novel action, be more effective than its predecessors and have no unwanted effects. Such discoveries are rare, not least because a medicine without unwanted effects has yet to be produced, and for the present is most unlikely. Although the risk-free drug will come eventually (we are already close with some of the vaccines and hormones), companies at present develop drugs with a careful eye to damage limitation. A product that causes severe unwanted effects will not only damage patients, but will also damage the company's image. Even an adverse report about a drug in an influential newspaper can knock the company's share price on the stock market. Bad publicity, like a drug's forced withdrawal from the market on safety grounds, damages profits.

As money-makers, drug companies are second to none among UK manufacturers. Over the last ten years total sales of medicines (on prescription and over the counter) in the UK have risen from £597m in 1976 to £2460m in 1986.[2] Moreover, during this period minimum allowable profit on capital employed averaged just over 20%. This is the lowest figure, the actual annual profits each year for many companies averages closer to 30%, achieved through the various perks and allowances offered by government as part of its Pharmaceutical Price Regulation Scheme (PPRS).[13]

The exact level of profit on UK sales is not made public. Drug companies are not obliged to say what they earn from the National Health Service in their annual accounts. The government, which sets drug company profits in the UK under the PPRS, knows, but isn't telling. These matters are commercially confidential and any civil servant who revealed, for example, how much profit Glaxo earns from the public purse would have been guilty of breaching the Official Secrets Act, and since the act was amended would now be caught by a new, but even fiercer, civil service code.[4]

Despite their coyness about the detailed financial picture, government and the pharmaceutical industry do release each year selected information. From this some of the grosser trends may be estimated. Accordingly, we know that during the period 1976–86 foreign earnings for UK companies increased by an average of 13% per year, (in 1986 it was £1536m),[2] while the number of people employed by the industry continues to rise and by the end of 1987 stood at 87,000.[5] Moreover all this has occurred during a period of worldwide recession, and in spite of the government's intent to reduce spending on drugs, a policy which culminated in 1985 with the introduction of the limited list.

Medicines and the City

The influence of the City on profit-motivated drug manufacturers cannot be overestimated. The banking community now employs specialist pharmaceutical analysts, themselves earning upwards £100,000 per year, who keep a watchful eye on the economic performance of individual drug companies, assessing profits in the light of drugs already marketed and those in development, making forecasts in the light of the prevalence and changing patterns of disease, and finally matching all these against company management.

Traditionally, the City's influence has been exerted along rather crude business lines with announcements of profit and turnover determining market dealings, but recent developments are now changing matters. The advent of the pharmaceutical analysts has made the city sharper and more sophisticated. But of course drug companies have responded by courting these analysts, and although sensitive to the charge (indeed, insisting that it is never done), may often attempt to manipulate their share price by leaking to them information about a new drug's prospects.

From the time the drug AZT (azidothymidine; Zidovudine) first came to public notice as a possible treatment of the Acquired Immune Deficiency Syndrome (AIDS) in the late autumn of 1986, to the time it was licensed for use in the UK in March 1987, share prices in Wellcome (the drug's manufacturer) increased by a startling 260%; from £1.92 per share to £4.98. But hyping by City brokers was not limited to potential AIDS cures. There was, for instance, also the market hype that caused Glaxo shares to rise by 60% over two or three months in early 1987, following the announcement that the company was developing a new 'wonder drug' for the treatment of depression. And why shouldn't the stockmarket be excited? This new class of drugs, if it replaces and expands the market made by older drugs, is expected to have worldwide annual sales of up to $8 billion.

Such links between the newly sophisticated City and the drug companies are not just one way – major management changes at Beechams in the mid 1980s seem to have been the direct result of City pressure. If this can be achieved then could not brokers silence those in industry critical of the City's influence. Examples of this are yet to come but I imagine Sir John Harvey-Jones, the former Chairman of ICI, may have been sailing close to the wind when he castigated the City for its 'fast buck' approach.

On a more optimistic note, it is just possible that the new intimacy between industry and the City could bring some advantages. The City might decide, for example, that indiscretions by drug companies may be counterproductive. It is not in the interests of investors if doctors, angered by the ethics of the pharmaceutical industry, start prescribing more of the cheaper generic or unbranded drugs. Share prices are also likely to fall if government, in the pursuit of economies, takes more steps to limit drug sales. If these measures followed overzealous marketing by the drug companies, the City could curb such activity. Attempts at this sort of influence are now being seen.[6]

Over the next few years the nature of the new relationship between the city and the pharmaceutical industry should become clearer. What happens will depend a great deal on the integrity and interests of the city analysts and one hopes that they will err on the side of morality. Perhaps the greatest problem facing analysts will be to persuade their colleagues that the pharmaceutical industry runs best on long-term projects with long-term investment. A search for quick returns could lead the City, with its new relationship, to strip the industry of its long-term, expensive but vital research projects.

A start could be made by introducing a more open practice,

with companies publishing more information about profits and expenditure.

In the USA, arrangements already exist to promote greater public disclosure of company dealings. For companies listed on the New York Stock Exchange (even the US subsidiaries of UK companies), the annual returns contain much more information than they do in London. The US regulations go even further; if the company's returns still lack information about particular facets of their business, then it is possible to lodge an enquiry through the US Federal Securities Exchange Commission. By this mechanism, it should also be possible to discover details about UK companies, such as Glaxo, because they are also listed in New York. It does seem outrageous, although characteristic of Britain's secretive society, that access to detailed information about a company must come by such an indirect route, rather than directly from UK sources.

Balancing Health and Profit

Patients must ask whether the pharmaceutical industry's success in business is matched by similar achievements in improving health. Unquestionably it has successfully produced many important medicines which provide enormous benefit. The prospects for patients with peptic ulcers, heart disease, asthma, diabetes, parkinson's disease, bacterial infections or schizophrenia have been improved out of all recognition by the introduction of new medicines.

To achieve this, money has had to be spent and outstanding scientists have had to be employed. To its credit, the pharmaceutical industry in the UK invests a greater proportion of its profits in research and development than any other manufacturing industry.[7] In addition, the scientists employed by the UK industry are in general of the highest calibre; almost without exception all of the leading academic pharmacologists in the UK are now working, or have worked, in the pharmaceutical industry. Furthermore, if cures are to be found for the many remaining diseases such as multiple sclerosis, cancer and AIDS, this sort of research commitment must be continued.

It is not of course possible to guarantee that major break-throughs will be forthcoming, neither, curiously, are such advances usually profit-led. If they were, drug discovery would be more common in the USA, where profits for the pharmaceutical industry are even larger than they are here. The record of American drug researchers in discovering genu-inely new compounds, however, is relatively poor. The real innovations require scientists of exceptional calibre working in intellectually conducive environments – in this situation the profit motive is rather remote. Sir James Black, the Scottish scientist who discovered the two most lucrative drugs in the world (beta blocking heart drugs, and the ulcer healing H2 antagonists) is just such an academic. He did not profit directly from his inventions, made while working for ICI and then Smith Kline French. What matters to him is the quality of his science, and he has a reputation for walking out of the door when his employers try to direct his research.

The larger multinationals have begun to recognize that the best brains wither in the hothouse of a commercial environ-ment. So now they buy into academic environments, either by creating completely new institutes within an older academic setting, as for example the Sandoz Institute in University College London, or by buying up existing departments virtu-ally lock, stock and barrel, as Squibb has done with the Department of Pharmacology at Oxford University (purchase price £21m, renewable after five years).

The chances of a company reaping commercial dividends from such academic investments are probably high, at least for the first few years. But I predict that innovation by the plundered departments will eventually slow as research is directed more and more towards commercial ends rather than led by curiosity, and as the pressure to guard company secrets undermines intellectual freedom. But when industry turns to the universities to replenish its research stock the cupboard might well be bare. The calibre, resources and morale of those left behind in the weakened universities will not be sufficient to bring on the next generation of graduates. It could be years before once--xcellent university departments can be rebuilt.

In an industry so concerned about its image, levels of expen-diture on research are now part of the currency of promotion.

As the rich in arid lands keep fountains playing during drought, so drug companies use announcements on research expenditure to advertise their success. In a single issue of *New Scientist*[8], three multinational firms announced their research spending. Bayer of West Germany headed the league with £500m each year, the French firm, Rhone-Poulenc, was second with an annual spend of £120m, and Hoechst, another big German firm, came a close third on £104m. UK firms seem to think that the sheer volume of their drug sales is a better measure of commercial machismo. In the same issue Glaxo boasted a turnover of £1,700 million and Wellcome £1,130 million. By any yardstick, drug companies are rich and powerful.

It would be wrong to suggest that there is never a streak of altruism in the behaviour of drug companies. The trouble is that standards and conduct in the industry are not uniform. Countless drugs are marketed in this country that are of no proven clinical value,[9] and some, such as the drug stanozolol (marketed by Sterling for the prevention of leg ulcers), might actually be doing more harm than good.[10] Hundreds are essentially duplicates of others already available (known as 'me-too' or 'me-again' drugs), while others are fixed-dose combination preparations, which are inherently difficult to use, can sometimes be dangerous and often have no rational support for their use.[11] Finally many drugs have been sold using inflated advertising and promotion techniques which virtually guarantee that they will be inappropriately or excessively prescribed by unsuspecting doctors.

But why should patients be used as the stepping stones to profit and why should this be permitted by governments? Of course people get ill, they need medicines, and someone has to pay to reward drug companies for their invention. But the ugly reality is that to drug companies, healthiness, or even a healthy attitude towards the use of medicines, is actually a threat. If by any Utopian chance, illness were to disappear, the pharmaceutical industry would collapse and the government would stand to lose its fourth biggest contributor to the balance of payments which in 1987 was just over £834m. In addition there would be the loss of employment for over

80,000 working within the industry plus the support jobs for a further 200,000.[12]

Such an extreme scenario is untenable but faced with an inkling of such a threat government chooses to side with industry to maintain the need and usage of medicines. To this end health ministers hold a dual brief: to oversee the provision of health while maintaining and sponsoring the industry. Prospering drug companies provide jobs and revenue; in such circumstances politicians go for the short-term option. But such a choice compromises any serious long-term investment towards a healthier society. If more time and money were spent on disease prevention, it would pay great health dividends in the form of fewer lung, breast and cervical cancers – not to mention fewer strokes and heart attacks gained from healthier diets and lifestyles. But the net result would also be fewer drugs sold, and, if one wants to be deeply cynical and conspiratorial, a growing population of elderly people would add catastrophically to the government's pensions bill.

So both the drug companies and governments have a vested interest in the treatment of illness rather than in primary prevention. Indeed the pressures on governments to keep the status quo are powerful, especially in countries like Britain where the pharmaceutical industry is such an important employer and exporter. The other big drug producing countries include the United States, West Germany, Switzerland, France, Belgium, Denmark, Netherlands and Sweden. Their total positive trade balance in 1986 from pharmaceuticals was £6,000 million.

Doctors are also compromised because they are inextricably bound up with the industry. As has already been said, most academic research departments, and many of the opinion-forming doctors and medical associations rely heavily on the industry to support their activities. Accordingly, the rare voices of protest that are heard from the medical profession are likely to be stifled or distorted by those who depend on the industry's largesse.

Useless drug proliferation is driven by the kind of greed and fear that propels the arms race. De-escalation of drug production will not come without a revolution in thinking led by patients and doctors. Only they can persuade governments

37

to restrain excessive drug promotion and to use only those medicines which are as safe and effective as knowledge permits. The drug industry must be compelled by appropriate incentives to target its research toward new therapeutic areas and genuine breakthroughs. This must apply in the Third World as well. Developing countries now buy around 20% of all drugs sold by the big pharmaceutical companies. Yet little research is done by the big companies on the endemic Third World diseases because those afflicted are judged to be too poor to make the investment pay. And now even the development of vaccines that are well within the technical and scientific capacity of drug companies is being curtailed because such products are seen as unprofitable.[13]

Industry as Paymasters

The pharmaceutical industry produces many more medicines than can be justified on clinical grounds. A typical GP uses only around 200 of the 4,000 prescription products available to him because his knowledge of drugs is limited and he does not see every illness. Many of the drugs available are mere duplicates of another product. Some, although approved by the authorities, are quite inappropriate. Others are ineffective and some are positively dangerous.

Yet the industry is successful in business terms, a position achieved by a mixture of ingenuity, expertise and cunning, supported by a penetrating public relations apparatus. Success has depended on currying favour among prescribers and politicians, quelling criticism when it arises, and creating a need for medicines and a climate of overprescribing. Somehow doctors, politicians, industrialists, corporate bodies and even patients must be made to believe in the industry's good name, in its positive contribution to society. They must see critics of drug company behaviour as unfair, discourteous, politically motivated – and where a UK company is concerned, deeply unpatriotic. Achieving this requires manipulation on the grandest of scales. Manipulation is most easily secured with money. The pharmaceutical industry has made itself the paymaster of medicine's decision-makers.

Pharmaceutical companies have given generously towards

the building and equipping of university and health service departments throughout the UK. Thirty one drug companies are named as benefactors on the commemorative plaque in the building at the Hammersmith Hospital that houses perhaps the most influential academic department of clinical pharmacology in the western world. Royal colleges and learned societies turned to the industry when they were originally established. Later they asked for help towards the development of new projects and fellowships, or to maintain college journals. The priming fund of £105,000 from Glaxo, Wellcome & Beecham was central to the establishment of the Royal College of General Practitioners in the early 1950s, while in 1985 £100,000 was given by the pharmaceutical industry to the Royal College of Physicians.

Examples of dependence are many. At present few if any postgraduate centres could continue to provide the essential lectures and seminars to keep doctors up to date without the sponsorship of the industry. Universities and even whole departments within the NHS are equally indebted. A substantial proportion of all medical disciplines, including less obvious ones such as surgery, microbiology or epidemiology, rely on grants from the industry. Indeed, an academic department not receiving many thousands of pounds each year in this way is unusual. As we have seen, the American drug manufacturer Squibb will now 'own' Oxford University's Department of Pharmacology up until 1992 (see page 31). It was the single largest benefaction which Oxford has ever received. Throughout the country, one-sixth of the staff of academic departments of clinical pharmacology, the discipline that has made itself responsible for evaluating drugs and advising on therapeutics, has its salaries paid by the industry. Salaries are just a start. An equal sum is handed over each year to fund research projects and any other extras which departments may require. Slides, books, and even journals will come free of charge with the compliments of the company. All the major prizes for academic achievement in clinical pharmacology are funded by drug companies. In addition, at least 60% of all medical research in universities and teaching hospitals is paid for by the industry, and the figure is increasing year by year.[14]

It is, of course, standard practice for drug companies to pay academic researchers for their services. But in some circumstances payments to individuals can be vast. Most of this money probably goes into laboratory funds and is 'legitimized', and it is in any case difficult to establish whether any cash goes into researchers' private bank accounts. But suspicions are strengthened by a report from the Royal College of Physicians on the relationship between doctors and the pharmaceutical industry. The report, which was published as recently as 1986, found it necessary to state that 'it is undesirable for a physician to have any personal financial interest in studies carried out on patients under his care'.[15]

Strong hints of diversion come from senior clinical managers within the industry who have noted with irritation a new wave of excessive demands for grants from academic drug researchers, many of whom ask that the money is paid into a private fund. But evidence that it actually does occur awaited revelations of the affairs of Dr Ian Robertson, a former senior member of the Medical Research Council (MRC) Blood Pressure Unit in Glasgow and a one-time President both of the British, and the International, Hypertension Societies. In November 1986 Robertson suddenly resigned from his academic post in the Glasgow unit[16] after it was discovered that he was receiving hundreds of thousands of pounds each year from the drugs industry. The donors included ICI, Janssen, Sandoz, Pfizer, and Merck, Sharp and Dohme. The payments were made for drug trials, for lecturing world wide, and for his many company consultancies; some were paid into his departmental account and it is alleged that others (upwards of £50,000) went into his own private account.

It seems reasonable to assume that these activities were undertaken with the knowledge of at least some members of his department, at least some of the drug companies and possibly some members of the Medical Research Council (MRC). Predictably the affair was not publicly investigated, and with the belief among his friends that his only sin was that of being caught, and that it was unreasonable of the MRC to ask him to repay over £10,000 of misappropriated money, Robertson was soon back in business. Within a year he had taken up a senior post with a large drug company abroad and he has continued to preside over international meetings on hypertension. He even published articles giving his address as the department which he had earlier left in disgrace.

The Vacuum Created by Government Cuts

The increase in research supported by industry is not the result only of pressure from industry. It has been aided by government policy to reduce public spending on research through traditional channels like the University Grants Committee (UGC), the DHSS and the research councils. When government began cutting funds the initial vacuum was more than willingly filled by industry, which jumped at the opportunity to direct further research to its own ends. Moreover, researchers, understanding company 'generosity', quickly learned that they could ask for more than they actually needed. Contracts from the companies, giving 50–100% over and above the true cost of the project, quickly became the norm.

At first both sides found this arrangement acceptable. Doctors could use the extra cash for other, possibly more interesting, areas of research. Drug companies presumably took the view that the more dependent the academics became, the more cooperative they would be if and when the need arose. But of late the doctor's demands for support have grown so outlandish that even the drug industry has begun to complain about the poor returns it is getting from its research funding in the UK. Several companies have even threatened to move their support for clinical research abroad.[17] No one doubts that there is still plenty of money available, but the quality of work being produced by the more opportunistic researchers was so shoddy that it had become an embarrassment to companies applying for new drug licences to market their drugs particularly in the USA.

Since then corporate purse strings have tightened. On the surface, this will prove helpful if it means that money is more closely targeted at the more able scientists. Yet, in a climate where money from both government and industry is shrinking, those who do receive funds may feel even more indebted to their paymasters, and then less able to express independent opinions on drugs and medical policy, than before.

The pharmaceutical industry's financial takeover of clinical research funding has another, and more sinister, consequence. Once industry has become the major source of funds, it can begin to manipulate the direction and flavour of original work and to determine the new data base, and can establish an agenda in which drugs become central to the way we deal with all ailments. Areas of medicine that do not depend heavily on drugs, or might even reduce their usage (like preventive programmes, surgical techniques, and even psychotherapy), will become marginalised. After all, their development might improve human health and threaten drug sales. Personally, I find the prospect of an insidious hijack of research as the most threatening challenge to patient wellbeing.

The Industry as Factmasters

The laboratories of any sizeable pharmaceutical company contain many thousands of drugs – that is, chemicals which have some measurable effect on biological processes. But very few will ever be licensed as medicines – those rare drugs which effectively treat disease without unduly harming the patient. Finding such compounds is difficult, time-consuming and expensive. Proving to the authorities that a drug is effective and safe means even greater financial risks, but also huge rewards. The most profitable drug in the world, Glaxo's ulcer-healing medicine Zantac, earned around £300 million in 1987 on worldwide sales of around £900 million.[18]

Before Zantac or any other new medicine gets on to the prescription pad, it has to be awarded a product licence. Strictly speaking, ministers of health are the licensing authority in the UK. In practice the real work is done by the Medicines Division of the Department of Health. Here a secretariat of civil servants sifts the mountain of evidence which supports the application for each New Chemical Entity (NCE), as prospective medicines are technically known. The decision finally to approve a drug as a new medicine is made on the recommendation of the Committee on the Safety of

42

Medicines (CSM) – a panel of experts chosen with the ministers' approval. In the United States the regulatory equivalent of the Medicines Division and the CSM is the Food and Drug Administration (FDA). No drug has a serious financial future unless its maker can win licensing approval in countries such as the United States and the UK.

The 20 year patent clock on a new drug compound starts ticking the minute that it is discovered and registered. But 10 or 12 years may elapse before the FDA or the CSM finally give their licensing approval. A drug company may spend, therefore, a decade or more and up to £50 million gambling that its drug will finally reach the market. The written information which a drug company must amass to prove its case from laboratory studies and clinical trials for a single drug is now so extensive that it can fill a lorry. In the early 1970s, a single bound volume of data would have sufficed.

The licence granted to a new drug does not give a company free rein to sell it on prescription. It also stipulates the form (tablet or injection) and dose permitted, as well as the promotional information which the company may use to launch and sell the product to doctors. Most importantly, the licence also limits the diseases against which the drug may be used, the types of patient (like pregnant women or children) that must be excluded, and any known side effects and precautions that a doctor should know before prescribing it.

The importance invested in this information is immense. Refusal to grant a licence invariably means that millions of pounds have been wasted, and *in extremis*, a drug company could be financially broken by failure. The sheer size of the gamble must mean that companies face a grave temptation to make the safety and efficacy data they submit look more favourable than they really are. Since the CSM and the FDA do not conduct their own trials on a new drug, they depend completely on the integrity of the drug companies they deal with. As it is essential for the collection and interpretation of these data to be impartial, one might suppose that the industry, the authorities and the medical profession would work closely together to identify and eliminate abuse whenever it occurs.

Unfortunately, the reality is very different. As we will see

43

controls are far from strict, abuses are commonplace, and the prevalence of misinformation is high. Over the years I have come to believe that this malpractice is undertaken with the tacit agreement (not to say collusion) of each of the interested parties – doctors, government and industry. But before we look more closely at the ways drug data are biased, we ought first to consider how drugs are chosen for development and how companies marshall their cases for approval.

The Process of Drug Development

The decision to develop a new drug is made by a company's new products committee, or an equivalent body. These committees consider the need for, and the feasibility of, developing each new product. They take into account the relevant disease statistics, scientific knowledge of the ailment to be treated, the alternative treatments in use, and the research facilities available. Each company has its own areas of research expertise or interest (hormones, antibiotics, cardiovascular drugs, drugs that alter mood and so on) and in these areas the company will tend to concentrate its research for new products. Occasionally a company will diversify into a new field of original research, but this requires a major policy change, backed by massive investment.

Companies do not produce drugs that come only from their own research laboratories, however. Since any innovative company can realistically consider developing new drugs in a limited number of areas, most companies will arrange other ways to bolster their sales portfolio. They may arrange to manufacture products under licence from other companies. Or they may direct research attention to producing 'me-too' drugs. Of the 47 new products listed as part of the clinical research programme of the US multinational Merck & Co., 16 were being developed under licence from other companies,[19] over 30 are likely to be 'me toos', and perhaps 5 classed by the FDA as true innovations.[19] Drug companies use three main approaches to discover medicines; they develop them from natural sources; they produce them by targeted research; and they find them by taking random compounds and screening them for biological activity.

Medicines from nature

The natural resources approach, which relies on a knowledge of traditional medicines and poisons, has been the classical way of developing medicines. It has produced drugs such as aspirin, (which was derived from the bark of the willow tree) the heart drug digoxin (which comes from the leaf of the foxglove), the muscle relaxant tubocurarine (related to curare, the traditional blowpipe poison of South American Indians), and the anti-asthma drug sodium cromoglycate, better known as Intal (which comes indirectly from the fruit of the Mediterranean plant *Ammi visnaga*). In this approach, substances are extracted from plants or animals, purified, and then tested in the laboratory to establish whether or not they have biological activity. If activity is confirmed and the drug has effects that make it a possible candidate for clinical use, its structure will be determined and attempts made to synthesize it and similar substances in the laboratory.

Learning how to synthesize the natural substance is important for two reasons. It gives the company a guaranteed and usually less expensive supply of consistent quality, and it also allows the company to patent its synthetic discovery. Until genetic engineering clouded the issue, it was not normally possible to patent molecules made by nature. Manufacturing patents can however be won on synthetic chemicals even if they are identical to natural ones. Moreover, drug companies often find that they can improve on nature by slightly altering the molecule to improve its clinical profile – to give it better absorption from the gut, fewer side effects and longer duration of action. By owning a string of very similar compounds a company stands a better chance, should the first candidate fail on safety grounds, of getting a new medicine to market.

One of the most exciting new developments from natural sources is the class of heart drugs known as angiotensin-converting-enzyme inhibitors – or ACE inhibitors for short. They owe their origins to the venom of the South American Pit Viper (*Bothrops jararaca*), whose bite causes local pain and swelling and, much more importantly, a swift and drastic fall in blood pressure. Brazilian scientists hoped that if this deadly substance could be understood and controlled it might prove of immense use in saving the lives of people with high blood pressure. They thought the venom worked by enhancing the amounts in the victim of a hormone called bradykinin which, apart from causing pain and swelling, also dilates blood vessels.

One of the Brazilian team came to London where he discovered the action of the venom to be more complicated. Although it did increase bradykinin levels, it had a more important second action. It blocked production of angiotensin, a hormone known to raise blood pressure.

High blood pressure, or hypertension, affects 5% of the adult population in the western world. Here was a potential drug of immense commercial significance, if only the active ingredient in the venom could be identified, synthesized to the right strength and controlled.

The US drug firm, Squibb, embraced the project. It took ten years to find and synthesize the active constituent which it called 'teprotide'. But even this drug was not of great use because it was made up of a chain of amino acids, which would be destroyed in the stomach before it could get into the bloodstream. Teprotide could therefore only be given by injection. Many more years elapsed, and Squibb nearly scrapped the whole project, before the first orally active ACE inhibitor known as 'captopril' was developed and given a licence in 1981. Sales of captopril reached $175 million in 1986 in the United States alone, and other ACE inhibitors developed by rival companies have also been launched. It was the enormous profits derived from captopril that enabled Squibb to spend £21 million 'buying up' the key research activities of the Oxford University pharmacology department.

Advances in the techniques for synthesising chemicals have been so swift that if Squibb had begun its search for captropril today its road would have been very much shortened. One such breakthrough has been genetic engineering which has brought renewed attention to natural substances. Insulin for diabetics used to be derived from the pancreases of cattle and pigs after they had been sent to the abattoir. It was a messy business, and not entirely satisfactory because bovine and porcine insulin is not identical with the insulin produced in the human body. Genetic engineers, however, can insert the human gene for insulin production into bacteria, which then happily reproduce in a fermentation tank, making as much human insulin as medicine could possibly require. No one, not even the most fervent of animal welfare activists, seems to mind if the bacteria have to be killed in batches to extract their precious product. The same genetic trick is now being performed on bacteria to produce human growth hormone to treat dwarfism in children, and to produce tissue plasminogen activator (tPA), a naturally occurring human enzyme which breaks down blood clots to prevent strokes and the recurrence of heart attacks.

There is now a major debate within the pharmaceutical industry as to whether genetic engineering, or advances in chemical synthesis, present the best way forward for new drugs. The size of molecule which can be synthesized has advanced enormously – but for the really big molecules, like the long protein chains of insulin, genetic engineering remains the best answer. Indeed, some medicines are still most easily derived naturally from the plant or animal where they are found. The heart drug, digoxin, is still taken from the foxglove, the anti-cancer drug vincristine from the periwinkle, and the anti-coagulant heparin, either from the lungs of cattle or the gut of pigs.

Medicines from targeted research

A second way of developing a drug is by narrowly targeted research based on what we already know about the body's behaviour. The human body has its own special ways of controlling its functions. Its systems are integrated, and run on information transmitted from one cell to another, or one tissue to another, by specialized molecules called chemical messengers. These messengers (also called mediators, chemical transmitters, or hormones) 'speak' to all cells of the body but only those with specialized 'ears' (receptors) pick up the message, and only those cells that can interpret the messages act upon them.

The hormone adrenaline is a typical messenger. Among its many actions adrenaline, which is secreted by the adrenal glands at times of acute emotional and physical stress, causes the heart to increase its pumping. After a traffic accident, for example, a burst of adrenaline is released into the blood which carries it to most of the cells of the body within a matter of seconds. Only those cells with specific adrenaline receptors, (of which there are actually four kinds), however, can receive the message, and only those with appropriate cell machinery can put it into effect. On the surface of heart cells, for instance, there is a rich supply of beta 1 receptors, and when adrenaline alights upon them, structures deep in the cell respond by making the heart beat faster and with greater strength.

With this information, it is possible for pharmacologists and biochemists to design and synthesize drugs to speed or slow the heart, as may be necessary in some conditions. The brilliant discovery in modern medicine was that of beta-blockers by Sir James Black. These drugs slow the heart if it is beating too fast, by blocking the beta adrenaline receptors. Subsequent experiments with beta-blockers have shown that they are also useful in the treatment of high blood pressure, angina pectoris, tremor, glaucoma, migraine, and, most recently, in reducing deaths from heart attacks themselves.

If Sir James Black could find a nearly perfect chemical agent to block the beta adrenaline receptors on the heart, it seemed possible that other illnesses could be solved in the same way. Sir James, the indefatigable scientist, was now bored with hearts so he moved his attention to stomach ulcers. Something causes ulcers to form. Everyone suspects excess secretion of gastric acid which erodes into the stomach or duodenal wall. Scientists knew that a natural substance increased the secretion of acid, so the search for a blocker that would prevent acid secretion, and so heal ulcers, seemed a logical step.

But ICI found this new area of human health too risky. Why mess around with the stomach when you are world leaders in the heart with propranolol, the name given to their market leading beta blocker. So they told Sir James that all they wanted from him was some improvement on his original breakthrough. A rival company, which had studied the patents, would soon develop a 'me-too' replacement for propranolol and steal a slice of the lucrative market. His first loyalty must be to reinventing an improved version of his original product so that ICI could stay on top.

Sir James did not much like this idea. His original drug was already proving a life-saver. Any successor was likely to be only marginally better. A new drug, along the same lines, to heal ulcers would be a real breakthrough of genuine therapeutic value. ICI balked at the idea. Sir James joined the US drug company, Smith Kline & French, which was prepared to listen to his novel ideas on targeted drugs to heal ulcers.

It would be nice to report that Sir James' relationship with his new company was one of perfect harmony, but it wasn't. Smith Kline, down on both its luck and its cash flow, came within weeks of cancelling the project when Sir James finally hit lucky again. Most drug researchers spend their lives never finding any drug of great medical value. In the space of a few years James Black found two – and not any two, but the two most profitable drugs in the world.

Sir James recognized that histamine, a naturally occurring and useful hormone, was the guilty agent. It is produced in one part of the stomach and stimulates receptors in another part to secrete gastric acid. He reasoned, correctly, that it should be possible to synthesize a chemical compound very similar to histamine that would fit into the histamine receptor sites in the stomach, but which would not activate gastric acid release. As a result the pain of an ulcer patient would recede, the ulcer would heal and surgery would be avoided.

Sir James' chemical discovery was called cimetidine or Tagamet under the Smith Kline trademark. It became the most profitable drug in the world until Glaxo, which had been working along similar lines, developed its close replica called Zantac which because of a slightly cleaner safety profile plus slightly greater marketing opportunism, has replaced Tagamet as world leader.

Sir James's new method of targeting drugs to mimic the body's functions has been nicknamed the lock-and-key approach and is now employed by every major pharmaceutical company in the world. It is intellectually satisfying for researchers and new computer modelling techniques now make it possible to design precision molecules likely to bind to the body's many receptor sites.

Medicines by chance

The lock-and-key concept, computer modelling, advanced chemical synthesis and genetic engineering make up the new approaches to drug discovery which herald a beneficial and profitable era for the pharmaceutical industry. But a third system still persists – the crude and tedious search for active compounds simply by testing scores of slightly differing compounds to see whether any have some biological activity. Many antibiotics, and even the benzodiazepine tranquillizers like Valium and Librium, were discovered in this way.

Medical seconds or 'me-toos'

If genuine breakthroughs, however discovered, bring great rewards they also expose companies to enormous financial risks. Therefore almost all drug companies spend a lot of their time playing safe. They try to find close imitations of their rivals' proven successes. It is the same commercial process that brings us almost identical pop music records, microwave ovens and low-fat spreads. Once a product is a hit, everyone else in the marketplace rushes to copy the original. Of course drug companies, like any manufacturers, have to avoid encroaching directly on the patents of their competitors. But this is not too difficult. The imitator may need only to rearrange a few atoms of the molecule that it wants to copy to skirt round patent law.

Making 'me-too' drugs has many advantages. The imitator does not have to waste vast amounts of time and money on original research. It probably also knows the imperfections of the genuine discovery and can hone its work to concentrate on the defects. The licensing authorities may actually appreciate this because they may be unhappy about some of the side effects of the original. So the imitator can even feel pleased that it is advancing existing therapy, at least a little. Once a 'me-too' drug is identified the imitator will still have to spend heavily on laboratory studies and clinical trials to convince the authorities that its 'new' version does work and has a similar safety profile to its predecessor. And when it does get a licence, the imitator will stress, in its promotion to doctors, each and every conceivable advantage that the new drug might have over the original.

The 'me-too' machine keeps drug companies busy and allows them to boast that they are working on a lot of new chemical entities, which technically speaking, they are. This pleases stockmarket analysts and convinces all but the most critical observers that the company's shares ought to be highly regarded.

Orphan drugs

A real problem of the 'me-too' mentality is that it leads to research excesses in some fields and because of limited resources, a research deficit in others. So while there are over thirty aspirin-like drugs available for the treatment of arthritis there are no drugs, and little prospect for any, for the treatment of sickle cell crisis, a painful, debilitating and often fatal inherited condition risked by over 5,000 mostly young people in the UK and many millions more similarly afflicted people in the third world. Why bother to research into the rarer inherited diseases or unusual infections when easier money can be made by producing a fourth 'me-too' to capture a slice of a large and clearly defined disease market? Why study the diseases of the third world, even though they afflict and kill countless millions, if the victims are mostly too poor to pay for treatment? The diseases caught in this vacuum have been termed 'orphan' diseases and the products which emerge to treat them, orphan drugs. In the United States a serious attempt to tackle the problem came with the Orphan Drug Act 1983. It encourages companies to develop orphan drugs by offering tax concessions on profits and seven-year mini-patents to guarantee sales. The FDA also offers grants for research ($2.8 million in 1986).[20] The authority also demands less detailed safety and efficacy submissions to reduce research costs.

In Britain there are ways to encourage research into the treatment of orphan diseases but these are mainly negotiated in secrecy. The Department of Health reduces its licensing fee from £2,500 to £150 – but against the total cost of drug research this is a laughable concession.[21] Privately, the authorities accept less thorough research on orphan drugs. By the end of 1986, 60 orphan drugs were believed to be on sale in the UK.[22] The exceptionally swift licence granted to Wellcome for its AIDS drug, AZT, must have been granted in this way, but this was never admitted by the authorities. Secrecy suits the government and the companies which are believed to be allowed extra profits on their ordinary drugs for doing good works in the orphan area. But as we have seen, the UK profits of drug companies are never officially disclosed.

Drug companies also shy away from research into areas which, although potentially profitable, could land them in court facing big lawsuits when things go wrong. For example, the Secretary of State for Health is now the legal licence-holder of 46 drugs, ranging from various vaccines to snake bite antisera and poison antidotes, which have been developed by drug companies.[24] They take whatever profits are made, but the Secretary of State orders supplies and, on behalf of the government, shoulders legal liability should the drugs, and especially the vaccines, harm the patient they were intended to protect.

This avoidance of risk lies at the centre of the conflict between a drug company's understandable desire to maximize profits for its shareholders and its obligation, perceived by the rest of society, to earn its money by genuine healing. This is also why so many drugs are administered as ointments, to be applied directly to the skin or the mucous membranes of the nose and mouth, where the chances of doing serious harm to the patient are relatively low, by comparison with drugs that attempt to deal with disease affecting the vital organs.

Genuine breakthroughs, because they enter uncharted areas of therapy, will always carry a greater risk of causing unforeseen damage to patients. All drug companies live with the fear of massive lawsuits resulting from the next thalidomide-type tragedy. 'Me-too' replicas ought to be safer since most side-effect problems should surface when the original break-through drug is marketed. This is not always the case.

ICI, the company that produced the beta-blocker propranolol, continued to develop others in the hope of discovering an improved version. By pharmaceutical industry standards, ICI enjoys a high ethical reputation, and it believed that the new beta blocker it came up with, called Eraldin, was without serious faults. But Eraldin was withdrawn from the market after it caused many deaths and serious injuries, including

52

heavy scarring to the heart, lungs and guts. The company was subsequently never able to repeat these horrible effects in any strain of laboratory animal. It would probably have won any lawsuit brought against it for negligence. ICI, however, to its considerable credit, waived the legal niceties, focused on the suffering caused by its drug, and agreed swiftly to set up a £10 million compensation fund for victims and their families.

The US drugs firm MSD faced a similar disaster after it won UK market approval for Osmosin, an 'improved' formulation of the anti-arthritis drug indomethacin. All aspirin-like arthritis drugs run the risk of causing gastrointestinal bleeding, but the company believed Osmosin was safer because it was designed to release its active ingredient slowly and gently in the small intestine. Osmosin was withdrawn from sale, however, after it was linked to the deaths of 40 people. The Osmosin capsule appeared to have a tendency to get stuck in the lining of the gut wall, where it released its contents locally in high concentrations causing fatal haemorrhages.

The Battle for Truth: How Medicines Reach the Prescription Pad

Even if all drug companies were always ethical and the licensing authorities forever vigilant, dangerous drugs which maim and kill would still reach the marketplace. Science is neither perfect or prescient and putting potent chemicals into people will always carry risks.

Moreover, the pharmaceutical industry has proved over the years that it cannot be trusted to behave ethically. In their rush to the marketplace, drug companies have persistently been caught exaggerating beneficial claims for their products and minimizing their dangers. This is why governments throughout the world demand that drug companies provide evidence of their claims before licensing their drugs. How good are the tests which the authorities set? And have drug companies learned with experience to evade or bend the rules?

Laboratory trials

From the thousands of chemical compounds in its laboratories a drug company is likely to receive drug licences for only a handful of products each year. Before any of these potential medicines is tested in human volunteers, it is examined in the laboratory and tested on animals. Unfortunately, most of these early data, which gives detailed information about a drug's behaviour in animals, are kept secret in Britain. It is known only to the company and the Department of Health. In the United States, however, the Freedom of Information Act allows anyone to scrutinize the laboratory records of a drug company.

In the UK we are unlikely to know much about a potential new drug until it is tried on humans – both healthy volunteers and patients – when most of the work is supervised by external doctors and scientists who publish their conclusions in specialist journals.

Healthy volunteers

Once an experimental new drug leaves the laboratory, tests are done in humans. For the most part these will be healthy volunteers (many of them medical students). Surprising as it may seem, there is virtually no formal control over these experiments. The volunteers are protected by no special legislation. The wording of the Medicines Act positively, if inadvertently, excludes them from any consideration. As a result, drug companies do not have to record or reveal who is experimented upon, nor are there useful guidelines on how healthy volunteers should be treated, and there are no specific insurance requirements to provide for volunteers who are killed or injured.

Official records show no cause for alarm. Healthy volunteers are normally challenged only briefly with a new drug to confirm that the effects predicted from the laboratory studies actually occur in human beings, to establish obvious side-effects and to find the dosage that will be needed to have the desired effect in patients. Drug researchers have long experimented by injecting themselves or swallowing their own medicine. In the United States, prisoners are permitted in some states to volunteer in return for money, extra privileges or merit points when applying for parole.

I have been a healthy volunteer myself on numerous occasions. I felt an odd tingling of the scalp when I took a blood pressure lowering agent called labetalol. And after being injected with a large dose of the anti-asthma drug, Intal, I felt a warm to burning sensation in the genital region. Inability to concentrate occurred while taking another experimental drug. But the most unpleasant response was vomiting in the London underground several hours after the study had officially stopped!

A recent survey by the British Pharmacological Society[24] showed that over a period of a year, in which 7,175 volunteers were studied, 81 in 1,000 suffered some sort of reaction. Most were trivial but in five per 1,000 they were judged to be moderately unpleasant. Two volunteers had very serious, life-threatening reactions. One needed emergency treatment for anaphylactic shock, the other surgery for severe stomach bleeding, after taking a three-week course of an experimental anti-arthritis drug of the non-steroidal anti-inflammatory (NSAID) class, which is known for this hazard.

In recent years at least two healthy volunteers have also died after taking part in experiments. In 1985 Philip Jones, a Welsh medical student, took part in tests on midazolam, a tranquillizer made by the Swiss company, Hoffmann-La Roche. Mr Jones died of a rare blood disorder several months after taking part in the trial. It was known that midazolam could cause the same disease, but since the disease occurs spontaneously in the general population, no proof of the drug killing Mr Jones was ever established and an open verdict was returned at the inquest. Roche offered the family an *ex gratia* payment; the amount was not disclosed.

The other recent death occurred a year earlier in the Irish Republic. The volunteer, Nial Rush, was given proxindine, an experimental drug for the treatment of irregular heart beat. It was suspected that the new drug's toxic effect was exaggerated by its severe interaction with a second drug which the volunteer was taking without the doctors' knowledge.

Although these two tragedies raised concern, at least in the media, the authorities have been slow to take action. The underlying reason is that the Medicines Act, which is supposed to protect people from the hazards of drugs, has no powers to protect victims if they are healthy volunteers. The Act specifically lays down that a medicine is a drug given to a patient for 'a medicinal purpose', that is to say treating or preventing disease, for providing contraception, or for inducing anaesthesia.[25] But the experimental drug which a healthy volunteer takes is not yet a medicine, because it has not yet been licensed as such. It is only a drug. And since the healthy volunteer is not a patient being treated for a disease, he or she is not covered by the legislation.

This is all the more absurd because healthy volunteers play a crucial role in the future licensing of medicines. Even though drug companies are not required to conduct tests on healthy volunteers, in practice it is unlikely that the authorities would approve the testing of an experimental drug on real patients in clinical trials unless healthy volunteers, acting as human guinea pigs, have been given it first. Yet Health ministers, who were recently warned by no lesser bodies than the Royal College of Physicians and the Medicines Commission, continue to ignore the problem.

Clinical trials: patients in the firing line
For many years a company could not test a new drug on patients in the UK until it had received a clinical trials certificate (CTC) from the Medicines Division. This required a full submission of the laboratory work, plus any healthy volunteer experiments, giving reasonable assurance that the drug will not harm, and may offer possible benefits to, sick people who have agreed to abandon conventional therapy to take part in the clinical trial.

Drug companies exhibit an obsessional urgency to market their compounds. In the early 1980s they began to complain that they were having to wait up to 18 months to have their applications for clinical trial certificates reviewed. They were able to enlist powerful support from academic pharmacologists for their complaint. The reason was simple. The drug companies warned darkly that they would shift more of their clinical trials abroad if the Medicines Division didn't speed things up. Suddenly doctors in the major teaching centres were threatened with a crucial loss of revenue from drug trials, and they joined the industry lobby. The Department of Health might have increased the size and the calibre of its licensing staff to cope with the backlog, but instead it offered the industry a shortcut; a clinical trial certificate exemption (CTX) scheme was introduced to run in addition to the CTC arrangement. Under the new scheme, only a summary of safety data from laboratory studies need be handed in, along with a solemn promise to report the outcome of long-term animal studies and any problems that arise among patients in the clinical trials.

It is only fair to report that the CTX scheme has worked well and has become so attractive to industry that the old CTC path is now rarely trodden. However it was introduced after unhealthy lobbying pressure, it reinforced the economic dependence of academic pharmacologists on the drug industry, and has been flouted in at least one instance (Sterling *v*. St Thomas'; see page 63).

Patients who agree to take part in clinical trials need as much protection as they can get. Up to 2–3,000 patients may take part in trials on a single drug which may last 18 months or more. Without successful trials, which establish that the drug appears to work and has tolerable side-effects, a drug company knows that it will have to throw millions of pounds and years of research away. Drug companies have every incentive to make the trials look as successful as they can. Excellent results obtained from a series of studies, all showing the drug to be better than standard therapy, yet having fewer side effects, will give a company a headstart when applying for a licence. They will also be invaluable as the basis for a promotional campaign once the product is launched. But even before that, the company can expect favourable reports from stock-market analysts to boost the company's share price.

In reality, however, much remains unknown about a drug until after it is made available to doctors on prescription. It was impossible to forecast that ICI's heart drug, Eraldin, would kill and injure so many people, even though it was tested in the laboratory on animals and underwent the normal clinical trials in human patients. Drug companies are therefore encouraged to continue studying their drugs after they have been granted a licence for sale, just in case something untoward turns up. Sometimes companies need no encouragement to carry on these so-called 'post marketing surveillance' studies, for the simple reason that they can use them to make money. If a soap powder manufacturer bribed a supermarket manager to put its brand prominently on the shelf where consumers were likely to buy it, we might not approve, but few of us would be morally outraged. But if a drug company set up a phoney trial pretending to test its drug, when it was really only bribing doctors to prescribe it over a rival brand, most of us would feel outraged. What a doctor prescribes should be determined purely by the patient's clinical need, and not by some perk which a doctor can collect, like cash, computers or a colour TV, if he or she changes brands at a drug company's behest. Yet post marketing trials have often been used for this purpose.

Post marketing trials can occasionally reveal some startling new features of a drug, which may make an unexpected fortune for the company, and coincidentally bring unexpected benefits to patients. The US drug company, Upjohn, had for years sold a drug for high blood pressure, called minoxidil, with limited success. The market has lots of drugs to lower blood pressure and one of minoxidil's drawbacks was that it could cause embarrassing hairiness in awkward places. Hardly surprisingly it was not long before the drug was mixed with an inert ointment, and rubbed on to the scalp of bald men. Some of them grew hair on the empty patch. Not perfect, lush hair, but hair all the same. The first genuine therapy for male pattern baldness had, inadvertently, been discovered. Upjohn named the scalp product Regaine, and is now expected to make a fortune from its windfall.

If drug companies carried out post marketing trials only to bribe doctors, or to find off-beat and profitable uses for their discoveries, they would need no encouragement to conduct the tests which ultimately improve drug safety for patients. But in most cases, these tests are seen as merely time-consuming and expensive, and drug companies have been reluctant to do them. Indeed, it has often required a grant or donation from a charitable medical fund, like the British

Heart Foundation or the Asthma Trust – or even the Department of Health – to spur companies into this kind of research.

The fact is that good scientific research, which genuinely proves a drug's worth and exposes its dangerous faults, is extremely arduous and expensive. It must be conducted with painstaking rigour.

Trial design: the 'random double-blind crossover'

The first test of good research is its impartiality. Neither the patient (or healthy volunteer), nor the doctor should know whether the recipient is actually receiving the drug under study. The trial should, therefore, be 'double-blind' to ensure no bias of expectation is added to the experiment.

Next, the recipients of the drug must be compared to a control group which is usually given a placebo (an inert replica) against which the experimental drug is evaluated. Alternatively, the control group may be given an existing, standard therapy to compare the effects of the experimental drug against its benchmark.

Both the real patient group and the control group must be selected at random, again to protect against any bias, intended or accidental. Ideally, the perfect trial would also allow for crossover – switching patients randomly from the control to the experimental drug and vice versa. They won't know when the switch is made, and nor will the doctor. All the records about who is taking what and when will be kept by an independent investigator.

This is the perfect world – a trial designed to root out bias and accident and reveal, by scientific precision, the true effects of any drug.

The real world is rather different. First of all, the patients available may not entirely reflect the many millions of people who will take the drug once it is on the market. The anti-arthritis drug, Opren, killed many mainly elderly people partly because they had lost their ability to break down the drug quickly and excrete its dangerous components from their bodies. Yet Opren was never thoroughly tested on people above the age of 65, even though arthritis is a disease which mainly afflicts the old.

Second, it is not always possible to use the crossover technique of switching trial patients from the placebo to the real experimental drug. It may work for drugs used against stable diseases like chronic epilepsy or high blood pressure where the symptoms are likely to stay the same for several months. But it cannot be used for drugs aimed at things like acute diarrhoea or a sore throat, where symptoms last only a few days.

Even the double-blind technique – the cornerstone of drug trials – cannot always be used. The anti-tuberculosis drug, rifampicin, for example, colours the recipients' tears and turns their urine an unmistakable pink. They cannot fail to discover whether they have been given it or an inert placebo.

Occasionally it becomes imperative in the middle of a trial to 'break the code', to find out who is on the real drug and who is on the placebo. This could happen if the experimental drug has a horrible, unforeseen side-effect which is suddenly discovered in some of the trial patients. It would be unethical not to find out immediately which patients were being put at risk. Or sometimes a trial drug might appear so marvellous that it would be cruel to deprive those on the placebo from taking it too. This happened during trials of enalapril, an ACE inhibitor heart drug (see page 45), when it was being studied in patients with severe heart failure. One treatment group in the study showed a sharp decrease in death rate – when the blindfold on the experiment was removed, enalapril proved to be the life saver. The same thing happened during early trials of the anti-AIDS drug, AZT.

Such breakthroughs, however, must be treated with caution, because drug companies have every commercial incentive to imagine a wonder cure when none exists. There can be no better way to get a new drug on the market quickly than to claim that to delay licensing the product would be to condemn those without it to death.

When antibiotics first came into widespread use after World War II, the US drug industry successfully exaggerated their safety and healing powers to such an extent that they won permission to add antibiotics to toothpaste and children's chewing gum.[27] Drug companies in both the US and the UK also overstressed the benefits of antihistamines as treatments for the common cold. Sales reached such a fever pitch that the authorities in both countries issued warnings about their excessive usage. Drug trials were then still in their infancy, but the then Ministry of Health in the UK was determined to investigate the drug companies' claims for antihistamines. It commissioned the Medical Research Council to set up at various centres the first carefully designed, double-blind, placebo controlled, random-order trial.[28] The results confirmed that the claims made for antihistamines could not be justified. And they established the scientific benchmark for all future drug trials. Out of these roots also grew the new academic discipline of clinical pharmacology which, in its desire to understand precisely what drugs do in the body, insisted that scientific methods must be used to test new therapies and the mechanisms of drug action.

This revolution in properly conducted clinical trials has spread to other medical specialities, but progress has been patchy. Cardiologists have embraced it fully and now use highly sophisticated techniques like coronary angiography and radionuclide scanning to measure the heart's function. But, for example, dermatologists (skin specialists) and otologists (ear specialists) have been much slower to adopt rigorous methods. As a result, clinical trials in these areas remain at a cruder level and inspire less confidence.

Publish properly or be damned: the importance of journals
The news media still have a bad habit of giving air time and column centimetres to wild, totally untested and usually bogus wonder cures. We have seen it with Laetrile, the apricot stone extract that was supposed to cure cancer, with umpteen fountain-of-youth elixirs that claim to halt ageing and senility, and most recently with various alleged cures and vaccines for AIDS. These stories are almost invariably put about by opportunists happy to profit by playing on people's fears and irrational hopes.

The major pharmaceutical companies do not descend to these levels. The scientific community expects them to publish the results of drug trials in patients in the established medical journals. The format of these reports, established in the 1940s, requires that the method of the experiment, and the results achieved, are described in sufficient detail to allow sceptics to make up their own mind about its validity. It also requires a clear conclusion, where the authors justify their interpretations. This standardized format makes it difficult to omit essential information without raising suspicion.

The medical journals are a firm backstop against malpractice, though even they cannot guarantee the truth, the whole truth, and nothing but the truth. The most reputable journals, like the *Lancet*, *British Medical Journal* and the *New England Journal of Medicine* require that independent experts, selected by their editors, vet all articles before they are published. No more than 15–20% of the articles submitted to the *Lancet*, *BMJ* or *NEJM* ever get published.[29] Some will be rejected because they are seen as unoriginal, but many others because they are scientifically flawed.

Sadly, however, the standards of some of the lesser journals are much less rigorous. They permit, for example, drug companies to pay for supplements which are printed in the standard journal format. Since these supplements are, in essence, paid advertisements, the journals may not always have editorial control over their content. But they look like ordinary learned articles and many an unsuspecting reader has been fooled. Subsequently, of course, the drug company will promote the claims made in these advertisements as if they were made after rigorous inspection by the journal's editor and expert advisors.

Self-preservation or Subterfuge?

One really has to ask whether drug companies are obliged to behave more ethically than other manufacturers of commercial products. If the maker of a new margarine or instant meal claims that seven out of ten housewives prefer it, many of us may laugh at the absurd claims and the gullibility of the public. What if a drug company, however, rigs its claims, pretending that its product is better, safer, more easily swallowed than its rivals? Can we afford the same wry smile? Yet drug companies do manipulate the evidence in the hope of putting their product in the best light. They choose who will do the clinical trials on their drugs, and it would be naive to think that they do not try to pick experts who are likely to give a favourable report. They also determine the design of these studies. So if the drug has apparent weaknesses, they may choose that it be tested in ways that are less likely to reveal the flaws. And since they are paying for the experiments to be done, they may also try to cancel trials which threaten to give unfavourable results.

Of course, not all trials are distorted in this way. But in my own experience about one in ten drug companies will demand of their trialists the right of embargo – to read, censor and kill unflattering trial reports before they are published. Why do academic doctors accept this censorship? Because, as we have seen, they so often depend on drug companies for their staff, for equipment, for travelling etc. Moreover in the worst cases they may be involved in academic or financial skulduggery,[30] even receiving personal kick-backs.

Even when clinical trials are conducted fairly, the drug company can still exercise censorship over results it finds unfavourable. It may choose to publish only flattering results,[31] and on some occasions selects only the favourable findings when it submits data for a product licence to the authorities.[32] The DHSS itself is currently investigating two cases where companies have failed to report serious unwanted effects.[33] Strictly, the latter may be against the law, although this position in the Medicines Act has never been tested. Short of snooping inside a drug company's laboratories, how will the authorities ever know if the results from unfavourable experiments have been shredded?

Why should a drug company behave so badly? The answer is that it can be extremely expensive to behave well. Millions of pounds are riding on a drug's future licensing and commercial success. Pressure has been put on the editors of learned journals by drug companies who fear an unflattering article may be published.[30] Alternatively, companies have been known to plant letters in the journals from sympathetic experts to refute any criticism of their discoveries.[34]

In December 1986 three senior cardiologists at St Thomas's, one of London's leading teaching hospitals, openly accused the US drug company, Sterling Winthrop, of attempting to harass and discredit them when, during clinical trials, they decided that Sterling's experimental heart drug,

amrinone, was neither safe nor effective.[35] They were threatened with legal action and in a final, high-handed act, the
Sterling company even arranged to have its drug removed
from the hospital pharmacy in the middle of the trial so that
the doctors were prevented from concluding their damaging
study. Even though the doctors were so incensed that they
made their allegations to a national newspaper, the drug
company, which denied the allegations, neither sued for defa-
mation nor complained to the Press Council.

Stacking the Deck

Trying to suppress bad news after the event is always a messy,
often unsuccessful, and sometimes extremely expensive business. Instead of trying to get the cat back in the bag, it may
be a lot smarter to choose a cat with no instinct to wander
into embarrassing places. Drug companies may be tempted,
therefore, to attempt to submit studies which, by their design,
will give a falsely low figure for adverse reactions.

Imagine you are a drug company with a new compound
intended primarily for use in elderly people, but you choose
to test it, instead, on people below the age of 65. The advantage is that your trial patients may not suffer the adverse
reactions you wish to avoid. Because they are relatively young
they are much less likely, after taking it, suddenly to lose
blood pressure when standing up. They will not have diffi-
culty in urinating or suffer symptoms of confusion. All these
reactions to anti-depressive drugs are common in people over
65 but are most unlikely to occur in younger test patients.

If this kind of deliberate 'deck stacking' seems fanciful,
then you may want to ask why the arthritis drug, Opren,
which injured 4,000 mostly elderly people in the UK and
killed as many as 100, was never formally tested in people
over 65 before it was licensed by the authorities? Yet it was
subsequently proven that many elderly people could not safely
cope with Opren because they were incapable of flushing its
harmful metabolites (the compounds it breaks down into) fast
enough from their bodies. The company's defenders claimed
that no one had thought to test drugs designed for the elderly,
on the elderly, in the days when Opren was being developed.

But rather than risk the embarrassment of an even more damaging court case, the makers of Opren, the US drug company Eli Lilly, offered British victims of the drug £2.25 million in an *ex gratia* payment in December 1987.

The trick may not just be in the choice of patients, however, it may also involve the design of the study itself. Most of the trials on the newer aspirin-like drugs, which are likely to be promoted for long term use, lasted for such short periods that the results were virtually meaningless.[36]

Another form of abuse is to exclude patients from a study if they are likely to develop a particular unwanted effect. This technique was used by Roussel, the maker of the anti-arthritis drug, Surgam, who were tried at the Old Bailey for making misleading claims about their drug's safety. All aspirin-like drugs are known to cause serious side-effects, including stomach bleeding. Yet in many of their 'safety' studies on Surgam, the company had chosen to exclude patients who had developed unwanted effects when taking other arthritis drugs of the same class. In effect, the patients chosen would be artificially tolerant to Surgam's own adverse reactions.[37] Later, we shall look more closely at Roussel's behaviour and the penalties which the court ultimately inflicted on the company and its medical director, Dr Christopher Good, for publishing misleading advertising claims based on other sorts of questionable logic.

Post-Marketing Surveillance: Prudence or Profit?

Once a drug is approved for sale, it becomes like any other product, from toothpaste to package holidays. Someone must choose it among competitors in the marketplace and buy it. One of the cleverest tools ever invented in this commercial pursuit is what drug companies call the 'post-marketing surveillance trial'. Since the adverse reactions of drugs like Opren, Surgam and thalidomide have been known to kill, pharmaceutical companies have an evident obligation to keep an eye on their products, and at least to publicize the problem and possibly even withdraw their drugs from the market at the first whiff of danger. How convenient, then, that they can use their watchdog costumes to mask their real commercial teeth.

In a post-marketing surveillance trial, a drug company will ask doctors to monitor how well their patients are responding to drug X, whether it is reducing the disease and whether it is causing unwanted side effects. Doctors are busy people, and besides, they may not, of their own volition, have put enough patients on drug X to give the trial any scientific validity. That can, of course, be remedied. The drug company will pay the doctor a small fee, or offer him or her a gift for the surgery, or possibly the air fare to a medical conference in a sunny part of the world, in return for putting more patients on its drug X. This is perfectly above board, of course, in the name of science and patient care. But the net result is that the drug company has effectively bribed the doctor to switch more patients to its own brand of drug in the name of good practice, prudence, and patient health. The value of the scientific data that comes out of these trials is often questionable, but their effect on sales is assured.

At one stage half of all the prescriptions written in the UK for the heart drug, Enalapril, came from a post-marketing surveillance study arranged by MSD, the drug's manufacturer.[38] Professor Bill Inman at the University of Southampton, who is the leading expert on adverse drug reactions in Britain, believes that nowadays these post marketing surveillance trials are almost always a thinly veiled excuse to boost sales. They are almost always conducted, he says, during the first few months after a drug has been approved by the authorities for sale. They are virtually useless in spotting those serious but damaging effects that occur only rarely because, in the early days, too few patients are on the drug. The statistical pool is too small to find a troublesome drug unless its damage is on a scale so great that it would dwarf all previous tragedies. But the trials are important in establishing the drug's market niche in the first few months after its launch, when brand awareness among GPs is paramount.

In 1986 the German drug company, Bayer, was accused by the *Guardian* of blatantly inducing doctors to switch patients to its brand of heart drug, Adalat.[39] The newspaper quoted extensively a former Bayer drug salesman who claimed that he was instructed to ignore all of the so-called post marketing data which he had been told to collect from doctors on Adalat's performance and side effects. Under no circumstances was he to send the data cards he collected back to Bayer's UK head office in Newbury, Berkshire.[40] He also claimed that Bayer had instructed him to reward doctors who played the game with cash, gifts and air tickets to foreign conferences. The Office of Fair Trading opened an investigation which was only dropped after the Association of the British Pharmaceutical Industry agreed to put its own house in order by publicly suspending Bayer from membership for a year.

These bogus trials are inexcusable, though they might be less reprehensible if the pharmaceutical industry at least paid attention to the real post-marketing trials that need to be done to protect patient welfare. Yet, in all the time that antibiotics have been on the market (some 40 years) we still do not know what is the optimal length of treatment for infections of the middle ear – a very common, painful and potentially dangerous condition. Why? Because drug companies have no financial incentive to pay for this valuable research. For the same reason we still don't know the real dangers of stopping a five-day course of antibiotics after the first dose, because the industry is only keen that we keep on taking the tablets regardless of whether they are needed.

These are just the sort of everyday problems that haunt GPs. They will not make headlines like heart-lung transplants, and the answers will not visibly save many lives. But a lot of people would experience less pain and cost the NHS less money, if GPs could rely on good, independent prescribing advice.

The Drug and Therapeutics Bulletin, published by the Consumers' Association and sent to 50,000 doctors in Britain, tries to offer this kind of commonsense advice. It also tried, in two recent issues,[41] to offer GPs a step-by-step guide on how to interpret the clinical trial reports so often influenced by drug companies. Market research showed that GPs thought the advice excellent in teaching them to find the holes in the dubious claims made for drugs. The overall standard of clinical trials are gradually improving but it is still common to read trial reports which have serious flaws which many doctors would be unable to spot. Once a medical lie is published, it lives on for years. The confidentiality clauses of the Medicines Act prevent even the most diligent researchers from getting at the raw data in a drug study that could expose a distortion or outright untruth.

The plain fact is that publication of shoddy clinical trials is clearly in the interest of drug companies. Worse, many appear deliberately to set out to litter the journals with waffle about their so-called discoveries.

Why aren't these carefully woven tales of deceit stopped earlier? The sad fact is that the medical establishment is nurtured on them. Doctors like the extra revenue they earn from post-marketing surveillance trials and have no incentive to ask whether they are valid. Even worse, many academic departments are kept alive by money they earn from conducting the pulp trials which end up published in medical journals. Their authors like to see their names in print. In the short term, publication helps their careers. The editors of journals also like to print articles which suggest that their publication is the first to report a 'new medical breakthrough'. They have no particular incentive to print an honest article which says that new drug Y is really no better, and arguably worse than its predecessors.

Ethical Committees

One safeguard against pointless or positively dangerous drug trials does exist. In theory, at least, ethical committees sit at every hospital or research centre where trials are conducted. They are supposed to have the final say over the safety and design of all drug trials before they are conducted on patients and healthy volunteers. They exist not only to protect the welfare of patients, but the good name of doctors and their institutions, and they usually include at least one lay person unconnected with medicine, along with a nurse, a local general practitioner and several senior doctors acquainted with clinical research.[42]

This is the theory. In practice things are, sadly, very

different. Researchers experimenting with new drugs in a clinical trial on patients have no legal obligation to get the ethical committee's permission before they begin their experiments. Even if the ethical committee is consulted, and finds the protocol for the trial inadequate or unsafe, there is no legal sanction against anyone if its recommendations are ignored.

The Medical Research Council insists that ethical committees vet any trials it pays for and the best journals will not publish results of trials that have not received the same scrutiny. But they are policing the quality end of the drug industry which in most cases behaves ethically anyway.

In the United States the rules are far more strict. The FDA insists that ethical committee approvals are included with all new drug applications. If they are absent, a new drug cannot be licensed for sale. In the UK, however, ethical committees can be ignored, and where they exist may be inconsistent, amateur and ineffective.[43, 44, 45, 46] For example, two thirds of the medicines currently licensed in Britain are identical to, or merely minor alterations of, existing drugs. Trials on these medicines are inherently unethical because they subject patients to unnecessary risks for very little gain, they waste vast amounts of NHS time and money, divert attention from real therapeutic issues, bulk up journals with verbiage, and inevitably confuse doctors.

Recommendations on the role of ethical committees when considering studies in healthy volunteers, were made in two recent reports to the government, one from the Royal College of Physicians,[47] the other from the Medicines Commission.[48] Neither seriously tackles the issue of how ethical committees can or could act to help control the excesses of the industry.

One solution would be for the government to introduce tighter legislation to cover the conduct of drug trials. As a first step, the Medicines Act should be amended so that substances tested on healthy volunteers can be classified as medicines. This would at least give healthy volunteers the same, albeit inadequate, rights as patients who agree to take part in drug trials. In addition, the government should make arrangements to ensure that the constitution and terms of reference of all ethical committees are similar, that no clinical trial can start without a committee's prior approval, and that the recommendations of such committees are enforceable. Moreover, in an atmosphere of these tighter controls, it might be easier for the government to guarantee compensation to volunteers in the event of injury.

But in reality the key to breaking the pharmaceutical industry's hold on medicine will not come by strengthening the control of ethical committees, but more by weakening the hold that government and industry have over information. Of course, drug companies must retain the right to protect their genuine commercial secrets from rivals and the government must reserve the right to control information, in extreme circumstances, which might induce unnecessary panic in the population. If all reports of adverse drug reactions were immediately splashed across the lay media, many patients might dangerously discard their medication without consulting their doctors. But the drug industry, and increasingly the government, use their power over information to protect their own interests and to hide their mistakes at the public's expense. Even doctors, who may be worried about the adverse reactions they see in patients, are prevented by law from examining trial data held by the Medicines Division, and do not have the right to publish data they have gained in DHSS-supported trials. Without far greater public scrutiny of drug companies' behaviour, the pharmaceutical industry will continue to use its carefully tailored facts to its own ends.

How the Drug Industry Cashes in with False Claims to Promote its Products

Until the recent cuts in the National Health Service we were, as a nation, getting steadily healthier. But for the first time in sixteen years, infant deaths increased in the UK in 1986 and 1987.[49] The AIDS pandemic has also cast a long and dark shadow over adult life expectancy which had, for generations, been steadily rising. Still, for most people the diseases of the past such as malnutrition, infestations, pneumonia, tuberculosis and severe bacterial infection have been conquered.

It would be churlish and quite incorrect to pretend that the pharmaceutical industry has not played a significant role in improving the national health. But now that many of the traditional diseases have been beaten, others even more diffi-cult to treat have taken their place. The emergent diseases like arthritis, heart disease and the cancers, tend to be progressive, prolonged, usually irreversible, and more often than not affect the middle aged and elderly.

Some of these diseases are self-inflicted, like the effects of chronic poisoning from alcohol and smoking. Some are the product of emotional deprivation, while others are caused by the eventual failure of the body to control the processes of repair and regeneration. Eventually all of these emergent diseases may be overcome. This though is the stuff of dreams and their demise is more likely to result from prevention than a chemical or surgical cure. The drug companies, however, would like us to believe otherwise. They weave a dream that cures are within our grasp, courtesy of their industry. And so long as we remain hooked on the dream, their commercial future will be guaranteed.

But reality says otherwise. There was a genuine boom in the development of novel drugs during the 1960s and early 1970s which brought real benefits like beta-blockers for heart disease, H_2-antagonists for ulcers, salbutamol for asthma, and L-dopa for parkinsonism. Indeed, the drug industry dream feeds off this golden age. But this era of discovery is passing. During the last decade many fewer useful new chemical compounds have been developed. Why has invention dried up? First, as we have seen, the diseases easily susceptible to chemical cures have been controlled. Only the tough ones, like heart disease, cancer and AIDS remain. Second, the cost of gambling on radically new discoveries has soared, while the window of reward has shrunk. Public demand for greater safety has extended the length and cost of drug trials. The extra time spent getting a drug to market also cuts down the useful part of its patent life: the drug industry in the UK claims that new drugs now typically have only six–eight years of protected marketing left by the time they are licensed.

This perceived squeeze has four anti-social consequences. It causes drug companies to play safe – to take smaller risks in well-established areas of therapy. It also encourages them, as we have seen, to cut corners on trials to get drugs to market more quickly. It also induces them to step up their lobbying on the Department of Health for big price increases on their existing products. And, as we are about to see, it spurs them to redouble their efforts to sell their drugs in doctors' surgeries with intense and often misleading promotional campaigns.

'Me toos': how old drugs are made to look new

Once a genuine discovery is made, like ICI's beta-blocker heart drug, Inderal, other companies will be quick to develop their own slightly different versions in an attempt to grab a share of a new and profitable market. The game is identical to that played by the food industry. Once one company develops pot-noodle or a extruded snack made from potato flour, the rest leap in with imitations.

The first 'me-toos' may have a few features which make them more attractive than the original. They may, like the anti-ulcer drug, Zantac, claim a better healing rate or fewer side effects than Tagamet, the first drug of this class. But subsequent copies, the third and fourth 'me-toos', seldom have much to offer except marketing hype and advertising revenue for journals.[50] In fact, they may even be damaging in the sense that they add to doctors' confusion and may cause them to switch patients unwisely from proven remedies.

This does not seem to worry the drug companies. By careful manipulation they create an atmosphere of fierce debate in the hopes that an otherwise irrelevant aspect of their drug can become the focus of medical discussion. Controversy is the perfect vehicle for embellishing a dull, imitative product. As minutiae are exaggerated so doctors suffer information overload and find it increasingly hard to make a rational choice based on the pharmacological properties of the drug.

More than £50 million is spent every year in the UK on over-the-counter painkillers. In one form or another, they are all combinations of cheap aspirin, paracetamol and codeine. If we all bought them in their generic form we would all get the same pain relief for a lot less money. To prevent this, the drug industry spends millions promoting their branded 'extra strength' and 'new and improved' painkillers which are nothing of the kind.

Similarly, we spend around £5 million every year on over-the-counter vitamins, yet few if any of these are required on medical grounds,[51] and for those in need the cheaper and more sensible alternative is a diet containing a little more fruit, fish and vegetables. Doctors write prescriptions worth millions for nebulous pick-me-ups and tonics, yet there is no evidence that they have any clinical effect.

Pain killers, vitamins and tonics, however, are just the small scandals. In 1987 it was estimated that 2% of the entire adult population of Great Britain (more than 1 million people) was taking tranquillizer drugs like Valium and Librium for anxiety or insomnia as part of their daily routine. In early 1988 the Committee on the Safety of Medicines finally issued a stern letter to doctors warning of the dangers of tranquillizer misuse and urging them to limit prescriptions in future. At the same time, alleged victims of tranquillizers started a legal campaign aimed at suing drug companies on the grounds that the seriousness of addiction to these drugs and subsequent side effects were not sufficiently warned against.

Now that the older tranquillizers are becoming increasingly discredited, a new marketing war is likely to begin. Glaxo, Beecham, Bristol Meyers and other companies are racing to develop a new breed of mind-altering drugs that acting by interfering with activity of mediator found in the brain known as serotonin or 5-hydroxytryptamine [5-HT]. Stockmarket analysts believe these drugs have a potential worldwide market worth at least $4 billion. While this new battle is being prepared, the drug companies continue to jockey for market share in known territory. Nowhere is this more evident than in the treatment of arthritis with aspirin-like drugs known as non-steroidal anti-inflammatory drugs (NSAIDs). Several, like Opren, Osmosin and Zomax have proven so dangerous that they have been withdrawn from the market. But new versions keep flooding on the market in hopes that doctors will prescribe them in the place of older, cheaper and more proven preparations. Doctors seem spellbound by all the hype: when the newer, but no better drugs appear, they prescribe them.

What real harm is done? So perhaps a few patients gets the wrong drug, and the National Health Service pays a bit too much if doctors prescribe a new, more expensive therapy. But another real harm is that the few genuinely new and important drugs, which should be licensed quickly, find themselves clogged in the same bureaucratic logjam as the 'me-too' medicines which the drug companies are so keen to promote. The Medicines Division of the Department of Health is snowed under by shoddy applications from the drug companies, so much so that its valuable work is impaired. Has this criticism been made by some anti-drug industry pressure group? Not at all. It was made in January 1988 by the two-man team chosen by a Conservative government to assess how the backlog of drug applications could be avoided. One of its two members was Mr Peter Cunliffe, the recently retired chairman of ICI pharmaceuticals – a man who can hardly be accused of wishing to impugn the integrity of the pharmaceutical industry.

So why are all these unnecessary copy-cat drugs allowed to swamp the system? The answer is that the Department of Health has a dual and conflicting role. On the one hand, it is supposed to regulate the drug industry. On the other hand, it has the statutory function of promoting the drug industry, and this means making sure that it remains a profitable portion of British commerce, capable of offering full employment and lucrative exports. How is this dubious circle squared? It isn't. One half of the Department of Health is trying to regulate the drug industry. It is trying to ensure that drug trials are done carefully with the patient's health in mind. The other half is trying to justify handing the drug industry bigger profits (through quick approvals of new drugs, price rises and sanctioning of 'me-toos') in order that the drug industry can continue to employ people and contribute to the balance of payments. Is there any sense in this arrangement? Obviously not. But Mr Cunliffe and his colleague failed to recommend the establishment of a regulatory agency separate from the Department of Health (like the US Food and Drug Administration), with the sole function of defending the public from the capricious demands of the profit-seeking drug industry.

Instead, we are left with a system which positively encourages 'me-too' drugs to guarantee that drug companies, now desperately short of genuine new discoveries, have enough profits to satisfy their obligations to shareholders and the Exchequer. Drug companies should be obliged to direct their resources away from trivial research, and back to the sort of invention that will genuinely be to the advantage of patient welfare.

Generic drugs

One way to force drug companies to focus on new discoveries is to take away the profits they are still able to make from their discoveries of yesteryear. This is easier said than done. Once a drug's patent has expired you might expect that other companies will rush in to produce their own cut-price versions, known as generic medicines. But the pharmaceutical giants use every ploy they can to squeeze profits out of drugs long after patents have expired. Have you ever wondered, during a trip to your doctor's surgery, why it is so often littered with memo pads, pens, and wall charts bearing the brand name of prescription drugs? Building up brand loyalty among doctors is extremely important. Hopefully he will respond, as we do, to television commercials, and scribble the drug's brand name down when he writes a prescription without even bothering to think whether a rival brand is better, or whether a cheaper generic variety of the original medicine is now available because the patent has expired.

As we saw in chapter 1, the government attempted in 1986 to force the prescribing hand of doctors when it imposed the limited list. This required doctors, in certain therapeutic areas, to choose cheaper generic alternatives when they wrote NHS prescriptions. The limited list should be extended to cover all therapeutic areas of prescribing. However, the savings are not as great as they should be. The reason is that the major pharmaceutical companies do all they can to deter generic manufacturers from legitimately copying their drugs. And, when all else fails, they also set up subsidiaries to make generic versions of their own drugs at the highest possible price to cash in on what profits they can.

Controlling the Dream-Peddlers

As a citizen, taxpayer and patient you might reasonably think that the government – through the Department of Health – cracks down on the drug industry's dream machine. In theory, it should. Strict rules are laid down to control drug industry promotion under the Medicines Act 1968 and subsequent amending regulations. The law requires that: drug promotions must not mislead;[10] they must be justified by verifiable evidence;[11] and every full advertisement to doctors must clearly and legibly list side effects, precautions and relevant contra-indications (pregnancy or other known conditions when it would be dangerous to prescribe a drug). Above all, the law says that ministers have 'a positive duty' to enforce these rules.

Are the government and its ministers doing their job? The blunt answer is no. By the early 1980s drug companies were flagrantly flouting the law in their advertisements, which made false claims for prescription products and failed, equally flagrantly, to warn of their dangers. Yet successive health ministers effectively colluded with this law breaking by failing to bring the companies to book.[52, 53, 54, 55]

In 1984, Mr Kenneth Clarke, the then health minister, admitted in a radio interview[56] that the advertising provisions of the Medicines Act had been broken 31 times in 1983. Mr Clarke said these breaches gave him cause for concern. But did he do anything about them? No. He said he would only prosecute when the breach was 'absolutely blatant, absolutely clear and where he thought he could get a conviction'. Instead, he insisted that his own civil servants and the drug industry's trade association (The Association of the British Pharmaceutical Industry) were effective in controlling abuse without recourse to the courts. Not surprisingly, the ABPI agreed that self-policing was the best way to deal with the illegal practices of its own members.[57] Yet research showed that more than half (56%) of full-page drug company advertisements breached the ABPI's own code of practice at the same time as these reassuring words were spoken. And the chairman of the ABPI, Mr Ron Wing, admitted on BBC 2 television's *Newsnight* programme,[58] that false claims and inadequate warnings etc. were so common in drug company advertisements that the entire industry would collapse if drug company directors were forced to resign every time a breach was uncovered.

In the pocket of the industry

False Hopes and Foul Play: Four Short Case Studies

Mr Wing was trying to give the impression that most infractions of the promotion rules are mere technical breaches and unintentional slip-ups, hardly worthy of a reprimand. It is true that drug companies produce mountains of advertising copy and innocent mistakes will be made. But let us take a closer look at four recent advertisements where serious false claims were made. Judge for yourselves the motives of the companies that made them.

Company: Labaz (Sanofi UK)
Product: Heart drug amiodarone
During the autumn and winter of 1983 the French drug company Labaz (which is known as Sanofi in the UK) placed prominent advertisements in one of Britain's most influential journals, the *British Medical Journal*, promoting its new heart drug, amiodarone. In bold print the company claimed that amiodarone: *Enjoys a wide safety margin and the time-honoured measure of toxicity (LD 50) is approximately non-existent . . . The side effects and contraindications seem minimal.*

What a splendid claim for such an important new drug. Yet in the smallest print of the same advertisement the following side effects were listed: nerve damage, tremor, photosenitization, skin discoloration, diffuse scarring in the lungs and hepatitis. These could hardly be described as trivial.

How can drug companies expect to get away with this? The answer is that doctors are busy people like the rest of us. They absorb big headlines, but don't always have the time or eyesight to read the fine print. In a study on an advertisement produced by the US drug company, Upjohn, 18 doctors were asked specifically to read the fine print. Six said they could not, without a magnifying glass, and the other 12 said they would not have persevered in ordinary conditions, but struggled through only for the sake of the investigation.[52] Unfortunately, there is no legal definition of legibility.

The advertisement for amiodarone, which was withdrawn after three months, was not merely internally inconsistent and misleading. A year before the advertisements appeared, the Committee on the Safety of Medicines sent its official warning

77

letter, called *Current Problems* to all doctors in the UK. It said, quite unambiguously, that doctors should exercise caution because serious adverse reactions to amiodarone had been reported. What is more, the reputable journal which accepted the advertisement had itself published an article warning of amiodarone's hazards,[59] as had the *Lancet*.[60] The later *Lancet* report, in July 1984, revealed that seven deaths had been attributed to amiodarone. We do not know how many patients will have suffered as a result of this advertisement, but I calculate if only 100 patients were put on the drug because their doctors believed the banner safety claims, then available statistics indicate that 50 patients would have become sensitive to sunlight, 30 would have developed tremor, 30 reduced lung function and 2 lung scarring.

The amiodarone advertisement breached the Medicines Act in two ways. Bold type information must be consistent with the data sheet supplied to doctors (Medicines Act 96, 3b), and promotional information must not mislead as to the uses and effects of a drug (Medicines Act 93, 7b). Yet the Department of Health, even though it must have been aware of the deaths and injuries linked to the drug, took no steps either to censure or prosecute the company. As a result, any patients who may have suffered will be unaware that they might be eligible for compensation.

Company: Eli Lilly
Product: Antibiotic Keflex
Drug companies are also adept at using 'knocking copy' – that is, warning of the hazards of rival drugs while claiming that their own are free from side effects. Eli Lilly ran a prominent advertising campaign for its antibiotic, Keflex, purporting to show that, unlike its rivals, Keflex did not cause severe rashes when given to patients. It pictured the face of a teenager looking somewhat apprehensive, 'Last week I felt like death. This week I look like it.' Brand X may be able to cure your patients' bacterial infection, but my goodness, think what it might do to the patient's skin . . . 'Nobody needs a rash from an antibiotic . . . try Keflex.' The sales pitch was clear. Other antibiotics might cause rashes. Keflex did not.

There was no evidence for this rash-free claim in the

published scientific literature on the drug. In fact, the official data sheet that Lilly had to supply to doctors on Keflex clearly admitted that it could cause 'allergies in the form of rash . . .' By law, the same side-effect warnings have faithfully to be reproduced, albeit in small print, in each advertisement. So where was the word 'rash' in the list of side effects that Lilly did reproduce in its Keflex advertisement? The answer is nowhere; it had been curiously omitted.

Company: Eli Lilly
Product: Insulin for diabetics, Humulin
Drug companies also like to play on doctors' emotions. What more compelling picture could they portray, then, than a young pregnant woman forced, because she is a diabetic, to inject herself daily with insulin, while she carries her unborn child.

Lilly is the maker of Humulin, a new, genetically engineered form of insulin which is designed entirely to mimic the natural human insulin which diabetics lack. On the available evidence, it is an excellent product superior to the older insulins which were extracted from the pancreases of pigs and cows. But Lilly's series of advertisements, showing the pregnant woman injecting herself with Humulin, clearly implied that she was sparing her unborn baby from the side effects which the older bovine and porcine insulins could cause. This is an emotive claim. It *might* be true. But there was no medical evidence for it. It breached the Code of Practice laid down by the Association of the British Pharmaceutical Industry, and was consequently withdrawn. Yet the advertisement still managed to win honours in a promotional competition, and the timing suggests that the advertisement was entered for the award after Lilly knew the ABPI was discussing its censure.

Company: Eli Lilly
Product: Anti-arthritis drug, Opren
The promotion, sale and subsequent refusal of Eli Lilly adequately to compensate British victims of its anti-arthritis drug, Opren, has been one of the worst chapters in post-war drug development. The market for arthritis drugs is huge. But all available non-steroidal anti-inflammatory drugs (like

aspirin, Opren and its many competitors) are known to have severe side effects, including gastrointestinal bleeding.

When Lilly won approval to market Opren in the UK in 1980, the company launched an estimated £1 million promotion campaign to convince doctors that Opren was a genuine breakthrough – an arthritis drug of exceptional pain-killing power which, unlike the other NSAIDs, could uniquely affect the underlying inflammatory process which creates the disease. This was quite a claim. No other NSAID on the market had any effect on the root cause of the disablement. What is more, Lilly told doctors that Opren had 'an outstanding gastric tolerance level . . . In fact the side effects story is very impressive indeed, as they are generally mild and transient in nature.'

The promotion worked. Opren was one of the most successful drugs ever launched in Britain. In two years GPs wrote 1.37 million prescriptions at a cost to the NHS of £13.5 million. But Opren's side effects were hardly 'mild and transient'. At least 70, mostly elderly, people are believed to have died in Britain after taking the drug and an estimated 4,000 suffered injuries which included gastrointestinal bleeding, kidney and liver failure, and extreme sensitivity to light.

In the United States, where Opren (under the brand name Oraflex) was sold only for a few months, Lilly's research director Dr Ian Shedden pleaded 'no contest' to Federal charges that he failed within the required period to alert the FDA of adverse reactions caused by the drug. A US jury subsequently awarded $6 million to a man, Clarence Borom, whose elderly mother had died after taking Opren. It is estimated that Lilly paid $50 million in compensation to all the US victims.

But Eli Lilly in Britain refused to admit liability and, because victims had to prove negligence in English courts, the company fought for five years to avoid making any compensation payments to the 1,300 victims and relatives of Opren sufferers who were claimants. Lawyers for the victims feared that any payments Eli Lilly might ultimately make would be small, because English courts have traditionally awarded only tiny sums (less than £3,000) for the death of elderly or child victims of personal injury, because they are not breadwinners. They were right. Even in the face of extreme public hostility (judged by opinion polls), Eli Lilly avoided a negligence trial by offering the 1,300 British victims a total of £2.275 million. This global sum for everyone was less than Clarence Borom was awarded for the death of his mother in the United States and amounted, on average, to less than £2,000 for each claimant.

The Opren case exposed the inadequacy of the English legal system, and demonstrated how cynically a drug company could behave when it knew it could escape real punishment for its promotional excesses. Had the case gone to trial, it might have been difficult to prove Eli Lilly's legal negligence in testing, promoting and selling Opren. But the court case would have exposed much which remains hidden about Eli Lilly's conduct, and it would also have exposed the role which the Department of Health (and its Committee on the Safety of Medicines) played in approving Opren for sale. The Department of Health was a co-defendant with Lilly in the Opren case. Perhaps it is not surprising that the Department of Health failed to prosecute the company for its obvious breach of the Medicines Act as it relates to advertising.

Why Government Fails to Muzzle the Drug Dream-makers

Ministers and their civil servants in the Medicines division have full knowledge of the abuses of drug promotion, but they choose to leave regulation to the pharmaceutical industry itself. We have already noted that in Britain ministers have two hopelessly conflicting tasks: promoting a successful pharmaceuticals industry, which presumably means allowing a steady and profitable flow of new drugs to reach the market; and ensuring that dangerous or ineffective medicines are not allowed to harm patient health or to waste the scant resources of the National Health Service. It is impossible, however, to satisfy the pharmaceutical industry's demand for profits while adequately safeguarding patients' interests.

During the first 18 years of the Medicines Act, from 1968 to 1986, the Department of Health prosecuted drug companies on only five occasions for advertising and promotion infringements. All were small operators working alone and making false claims for products sold on a small scale. It seemed that the department was not prepared to confront large drug companies, even though their promotional breaches, as we have seen, are often flagrant. Nor is the department eager to limit the scale of the promotional hype of the drugs industry: more than £180 million is spent each year convincing British doctors to prescribe medicines. By contrast, the department spends only £4 million a year providing impartial advice on drug usage to GPs and hospital doctors.

What about the industry's own, self-appointed regulators, the code of practice committee at the Association of the British Pharmaceutical Industry? The committee is a watchdog with virtually no bark and certainly no teeth. It has no legal status, no enforceable sanctions, and its secret deliberations offer no public accountability. Indeed, like many critics, I assume that its primary role is to shield the pharmaceutical industry from the public scrutiny of the law courts. Furthermore, the code of practice committee does not even require drug companies to submit their advertisements for vetting before publication. It thus cannot prevent misleading advertisements from appearing, and over the years has only acted after a complaint from a doctor or a competing drug company. By the time it finishes its deliberations (which usually take several months) a drug company's promotional campaign will already have achieved its ends and patients may have suffered.

Punishment too is pitiful. A drug company which breaches the code can expect no more reprimand than a brief mention of its misbehaviour in selected medical journals, and a request that the advertisement be withdrawn.

The only effective way to deal with misleading advertisements is to prevent them from ever appearing, and the only way to do that is to ensure that where there is a serious breach then the company concerned risks prosecution under the Medicines Act. In December 1985, the Department of Health began its first criminal prosecution of a major drug company.[61] The case against the company Roussel, its verdict and its implications deserve close scrutiny.

Crown v. Roussel, the Old Bailey, December 1985

Roussel is one of the biggest drug companies in Europe. It is heavily influenced by its largest shareholder, Hoechst of West Germany, the leading pharmaceutical company in Europe. In 1982 Roussel won permission to market Surgam, its brand of anti-arthritis drug, in Britain. With hindsight, Surgam or tiaprofenic acid, has proved to be typical of the non-steroidal anti-inflammatory class of pain killers prescribed for arthritis sufferers. None of the NSAIDs can get to the root cause of the disease to arrest its destruction of the joints, and all the NSAIDs can cause gastrointestinal bleeding as well as other side effects. Roussel was not content merely to slot Surgam into the highly lucrative, but already overcrowded arthritis drug market. The company was looking for a unique selling point that would convince doctors to switch their arthritis patients to Surgam. As we are about to see, it was very successful. There was no evidence that Surgam could attack the root causes of arthritis. Roussel claimed in its advertising that Surgam was much gentler on the stomach than its rivals because it, uniquely had 'selective prostaglandin inhibition'. Prostaglandins are a diverse group of compounds made by the body which have very different functions. Prostaglandins E and F stimulate the pain-sensitive nerve endings, which causes the brain to feel pain. All the NSAID arthritis drugs work by suppressing the production of these prostaglandins to a greater or less extent. A third type, prostaglandin I, has yet other actions, one of which is to protect the stomach lining against ulcer formation. Since the NSAIDs block the formation of all three equally, any NSAID that relieves pain is also likely to cause bleeding in the stomach. Roussel decided to claim that Surgam, unlike its rivals, 'had far less effect' on prostaglandin I in the stomach, and therefore it was safer to use.

In four separate advertisements published in the *British Medical Journal* between March and June 1983, Roussel claimed in large, bold print for Surgam that it offered not only 'tolerance in the stomach', but even 'gastric protection'. Buried in the small print, however, Roussel admitted that Surgam should be used 'with care in patients with a history of peptic ulceration' – as it was required to do by the Commiitee on the Safety of Medicines when granted its product licence to market Surgam. But if Surgam was a potential danger to ulcer patients, how could it legitimately confer 'gastric protection' on anyone? Here was a suspected case of misleading advertising so gross that even the Department of Health could not ignore it.

Criminal proceedings began at the Central Criminal Court in December 1985. The company faced two charges under the Medicines Act: that its advertisement 'was misleading in that the claims for gastric protection and selective prostaglandin inhibition were not justified or substantiated by clinical or other appropriate trials or studies'. The second charge, relating to Roussel's particular claim that Surgam was safer than a rival arthritis drug, indomethacin, was later dropped. Also in the dock, and personally charged with the alleged offences was Roussel's medical director, Dr Christopher Good, who is, in law, responsible for promotional claims made by the company.

The case lasted four weeks and the long-suffering jury was subjected to long submissions from expert witnesses on prostaglandin synthesis and on pharmacology. Much of the evidence was so abstruse and dull that someone posted a hand written sign on the door of the public gallery which read, 'Chemical fraud – very boring', to warn passers by to choose a rape or murder trial in another court instead.

Almost buried in this welter of detail was the crucial issue: what evidence did Roussel really have to justify its claim that Surgam, unlike all other arthritis drugs, offered 'gastric protection' by sparing the protective prostaglandin I in the stomach? Had the company demonstrated this crucial effect in the stomachs of humans in clinical trials? Had it at least proven the benefits of Surgam in the stomachs of live animals? No, neither. The only evidence Roussel could produce was from experimental studies on two animal tissues (neither of which were stomach tissue) which they had combined in order to support their claim.

Even the expert witnesses called by Roussel in its defence, Professor Paul Turner and Professor Rod Flower, testified that data from animals could not be extrapolated safely to patients. Roussel concocted its claim by transforming a highly theoretical hypothesis from the laboratory into a dogmatic statement to be read and believed by doctors in the *British Medical Journal*. Internal Roussel memoranda disclosed to the court even showed that many of the company's own consultants never believed the gastric protection claim. One crucial memo showed that even the company, and Dr Good personally, had accepted that the basis of the claim was untenable the day before the first advertisement appeared on March 26.

Roussel and Dr Good were found guilty of making misleading claims for Surgam in the April, May, and June advertisements which appeared in the *British Medical Journal*. They were acquitted of making misleading claims in the March advertisement, presumably because it appeared so soon after the internal memo and its publication could not have been stopped. Roussel was fined £20,000 and ordered to pay net costs of £23,800. Dr Good was fined £1,000 although his own costs were covered by the Medical Defence Union, the mutual insurance fund for doctors.[62] The fines were paltry considering the assets and profits of a company as large as Roussel. In 1986 it spent £415,195 just on advertising Surgam, which remains on the market.

Roussel and Dr Good lodged an appeal which was heard in May 1988. They recognized that their advertisement had been misleading in that it had not reflected current knowledge at the time of publication, but argued that their misdemeanour was not caught by the law. The breach, they said, could not be described in terms of the drug's 'nature or quality, uses or effects', and this would have to be so if it were to be found misleading under the Medicines Act. Obviously the meaning of these words, particularly that of 'quality', was crucial and the appellants argued that in the original proceedings the judge had misdirected the jury as to their definition. The appeal was dismissed.

During the appeal, as at the original hearing, counsel for Roussel and Good tried to present their offence as trivial. This notion too the judges dismissed.[63] Dr Good may now have to appear before the General Medical Council which has powers to strike his name from the medical register.

The case against Roussel also has wide implications for the

drug industry, doctors and patients. Before it, drug companies must have regarded the risk of prosecution as remote – an acceptable gamble in return for a successful promotional campaign to boost drug sales and profits. Now, at least, the odds have shortened. Medical directors in other companies, knowing that they could be threatened by criminal prosecution, may help in future to maintain more honest and ethical drug promotion. They may be able to wrest some of the power within the industry away from its marketing departments.

Misleading advertising, however, is only the visible part of a complex network of illicit influence wielded by the pharmaceutical industry. There are no effective laws governing the way drug companies use their lobbying influence to win favour with politicians and other opinion formers. Whitehall officials, who set drug company profits under the Pharmaceuticals Price Regulation Scheme (PPRS), are given a clue when they ask to see how much individual companies spend on promotion. Money spent on influencing doctors with gifts, favours, bogus drug trials and research seminars is easily disguised as research expenditure. And no revelations are ever made public – these negotiations with Whitehall are official secrets.

The behaviour of the pharmaceutical industry places both doctors and patients in jeopardy. If doctors believe all drug industry claims, then patients must surely suffer. On the other hand, an atmosphere of mistrust may also deny patients genuinely useful and effective therapies.

Doctors and patients are striving for one thing: health. But the pharmaceutical industry is pressing just as hard for profits. In a disease-free society, the pharmaceutical industry would be superfluous. Just as undertakers thrive on death, so the pharmaceutical industry thrives on disease. Making a profit at the expense of patients' health is indefensible. It would seem, however, that the government, which ought to defend both doctors and patients from the flagrant abuses of the drug industry, is failing manifestly to do its duty.

No doubt the government will point to its successful prosecution of Roussel in the Surgam case as a measure of its vigilance. Those who believe this will be misled on two counts. I spent many days at the Old Bailey watching the

Roussel case unfold and I firmly believe that it was grossly mishandled and very nearly lost because influential people within Whitehall and government never wanted the case to come to trial in the first place. For such an important test case, experts from the medicines division of the Department of Health, with wide knowledge both of arthritis drugs and drug industry promotion, should have been available to assist the prosecution lawyers. Instead, the government offered a relatively minor official who no longer worked in the relevant fields. And even though the government had nearly two years to prepare its case against Roussel, it was still seeking crucial advisers and expert witnesses when the case was near to trial. Moreover, if the government seriously wanted to stop the promotional abuses of the pharmaceutical industry, it would not need to spend time and taxpayers' money tortuously fighting drug companies in court. The fact is that ministers have direct powers under the Medicines Act to prohibit dubious promotions and advertisements immediately. But it fails to use them and so puts the interests of the pharmaceutical industry before the welfare of patients.

CHAPTER 3

Government: The Double Agent

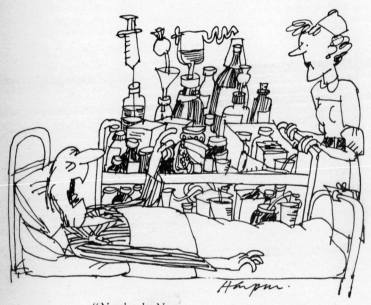

"No thanks Nurse—
I'll just take the 3 million pounds."

CHAPTER 3

Government: The Double Agent

On the day that we, or our loved ones, fall ill the National Health Service becomes very personal. It is no longer a vast bureaucracy. We expect it, quite reasonably, to work well for us because our lives are at stake. We have paid, through National Insurance contributions, for the privilege of care. But the truth is that, as individuals, we can demand next to nothing. The very Act that established the National Health Service in 1948 says nothing about *individual* rights (1). It talks only about the obligation to establish 'a comprehensive health service designed to secure the improvement in the physical and mental health of the *people* . . .'. More recently the DHSS recognized that the health service should provide 'guaranteed commitment for improvement in services and concern for the well-being of every individual patient'.[2] 'Improvements' and 'concern' are welcome but the 1946 position remains unchanged – the DHSS offers nothing tangible to the individual claiming his or her rights.

Individual demands on the health service, if added together, are insatiable. The cruel reality is that the government has to make choices. The government is, therefore, a double agent. It has to balance escalating demands of patients against the cost to the general public of treating the sick.

The Thatcher government's answer to this dilemma has been uncompromising. Health care is expected to run on a shoestring. Government is now allocating around £21 billion to the NHS and an additional £2 billion is spent on private health care. Large as these figures may seem, they add up to far less than any other country of equivalent wealth spends on the health of its people. The facts of health in Britain speak for themselves. Infant mortality, after a long and steady fall, is now rising again.[3] Life expectancy for forty-year-olds (the next age group at which figures begin again to reflect health provision) is now shorter in Britain than it is almost anywhere else in the developed world.[4, 5]

Our health record is lamentable because ministers have *chosen* to let health spending fall, in real terms, at a time when the national wealth is rising. By stealth, the national health is being abused.

If demand for health care exceeds supply, is it because demand is insatiable, or because the supply is unjustifiably restricted? There is a very real difference between the two cases. Was it really necessary, owing to insatiable demand, to allow four Midlands children, Matthew Collier, Nathan Bates, David Barber and Scott Kimberley[6] to die in 1988 from heart disease in circumstances which strongly suggested that their deaths might have been avoided, or at least that their suffering might have been reduced, had adequate health provision been offered by the cash-starved local authority?

Ministers did nothing to help. They had, for political reasons, engineered the circumstances which forced these children to face long waiting-list delays, last minute cancellations, and arguably their premature deaths. Insatiable demands are nevertheless real. Diabetic patients who happen to live near to a specialist ophthalmic hospital may have their sight saved by costly ophthalmic laser surgery. Others, less fortunate, will become blind, a common outcome of this illness. There cannot be specialist centres for all diseases in every locality. Choices have to be made. Heart transplants will take money from kidney dialysis. Many might choose to restore useful life to transplant patients even if it means allowing elderly renal patients to die. But lines must be drawn, compassion felt and ultimately, paid for. In any affluent and civilized society it is disgraceful that elderly people, otherwise healthy but in great pain, should have to wait years for a hip replacement or a hernia repair. Yet this is commonplace and has become government policy.

There is also a fundamental difference between knowing that some people may die and choosing, parsimoniously, to let many die. The whooping cough vaccine, for all its controversial limitations, benefits the general population – a view upheld by the High Court in March 1988. Rare children, sensitive to it, may suffer brain damage and even death. This is a terrible toll and a better vaccine must be developed. But life without the vaccine would be worse, because an even greater number of children would die or be permanently handicapped by the disease if the vaccine did not exist.

Health is a Political Issue

By allocating money, the government chooses the kind of medicine it will support. It decides the number and quality of future doctors by funding the University Grants Committee. It controls the career structures, salaries and numbers of serving doctors in general practice and in the hospital service by decree and by careful cultivation of the various Royal Colleges. It decides the hospital spending of each region, the number of beds allocated to each specialty – even the number of nurses and clinics – through its political appointees in the Regional Health Authorities. It is no coincidence that 13 of the 14 authorities are chaired by members of the Conservative Party.

Even so, medicine is expensive and difficult to manage. The NHS with 1.3 million staff spends nearly £15 billion on salaries and wages.[7] By contrast, £2 billion spent on drugs appears cheap. Drugs have reduced disease and death. They do cut the number of days people must remain expensively in hospital. And they are produced by companies which are unswervingly loyal, and often munificent contributors, to the Conservative party (£100,000 in 1986).[8]

All political parties in power, mindful of the drug industry's influence, and its role as an employer and exporter, are loathe to anger it. Are governments, of any colour, capable of controlling and regulating it?

The Politics of Drugs

The cost of most health provision is tightly controlled. The government ultimately decides how many hospitals to build, how many doctors to train, and how many nurses to employ. But it has very little control over the drugs bill. General practitioners largely have a blank cheque to prescribe what they will. The cheques are paid when the prescriptions written up and down the country wend their way to the Prescription Pricing Authority in Newcastle.

Why is the doctor's right to prescribe virtually sacrosanct? There are two fundamental reasons. It is still believed (with the exception of the limited list) that the state should not intrude upon the intimate relationship between doctors and patients. Doctors know best which drugs will make their patients well. Secondly, governments remain convinced, for reasons already explained, that they are getting a bargain from medicines. They do save lives, and in crude cash terms they do cut down on expensive treatment. Even Labour governments have been reluctant, therefore, to interfere in drugs policy.

This is a naïve view, as the thalidomide disaster, and later, the Opren tragedy, proved. Doctors can become the gullible victims of drug company promotion. They prescribed thalidomide to pregnant women because they were told by Distillers (the makers of the sleeping tablet) that it was safe to do so. We all know the consequences of this terrible misinformation. Doctors were told, with equal force, that Opren was an excellent and safe drug for the control of arthritis in the elderly. It was only 20 years ago, however, in the wake of the thalidomide disaster, that the Medicines Act (1968) was passed to regulate drug licensing and prescribing. Before then, only vague legislation existed and the drugs industry was left, virtually, to regulate itself. The thalidomide tragedy shocked governments around the world. The Medicines Act followed a detailed enquiry into drug company profits and promotion known as the Sainsbury Report.[9]

Essentially, the Act did two things. It established a Medicines Commission which is charged with advising ministers on all matters of drugs policy. It also established a Medicines Division within the Department of Health which has the day to day job of licensing new drugs, overseeing their use, and reviewing whether their dangers, once in use, outweigh their benefits.

The Medicines Commission has a variable composition, and in 1987 consisted of 24 members chosen by the Secretary of

State for Health, of whom ten were conventionally trained doctors and the remainder included pharmacists, chemists, veterinary surgeons, laboratory scientists, lawyers and one specialist in holistic medicine. Of the membership, five came from the pharmaceutical industry.

The Medicines Division, however, is the real working engine of drugs control. It has five committees concerned with drug use in patients, and all are appointed by the minister. The most important is the Committee on Safety of Medicines (CSM) which recommends to ministers whether *new* drugs should be licensed for sale and whether drugs subsequently proven dangerous should be withdrawn. The Committee on the Review of Medicines (CRM), has the job of reviewing and licensing the *old* drugs that were already available when the medicines act was first introduced. Members of the Committees are not civil servants. They are medical experts from clinical practice, the industry and the universities who come regularly to London to perform their part-time advisory role. They are served by a team of about 300 civil servants within the division.

The Committee on Safety of Medicines captures most of the headlines. It came under attack for failing, more quickly, to spot the dangers of Opren and some of the other dangerous anti-arthritis drugs. More recently, the CSM warned all doctors to take greater care in prescribing tranquillizers like Valium and Ativan,[10] at a time when allegedly dependent patients began to mount lawsuits against their doctors and the drug manufacturers. But the Committee on the Review of medicines also has an important, if often overlooked role. It has had to plough laboriously through the 39,000 drug preparations which were already on the market before the CSM was established. The CRM was established in 1975. By the following year the drug companies chose to withdraw around 10,000 of these products after they were assked by the CRM to submit comprehensive information proving their worth. One can only assume that this headlong exodus happened because the drug companies knew that support for their products was flimsy in the extreme and they feared public ridicule if it became known that they had marketed worthless, and even dangerous, products. Since then the CRM has annually called for the review of around 3,000 drugs – and each year about half are 'voluntarily' withdrawn from sale by drug companies unwilling to see their products subjected to such scrutiny. By 1990 this job will have been completed and the CRM disbanded.

The Dual Role of the Double Agent

Such a regime may seem tough and vigilant, but the drug companies continue to get away with marketing and profiting from drugs for which patients have no real need. We have already seen that ministers at the Department of Health have a dual role. This dilemma could be solved in one of two ways. Either, the Department of Trade and Industry could take over the role of 'sponsoring' the drug industry,[11] or the regulation of drugs and drug companies could be hived off into a separate agency, like the Food and Drug Administration in the United States. But both these calls for reform have been ignored. Kenneth Clarke, during his first term as Health Minister, let his embarrassment at having to sponsor the pharmaceutical industry be known. But he failed to persuade his ministerial colleagues to transfer the sponsorship role to the Department of Trade and Industry.

The pharmaceutical industry works hard to make sure that its views are represented. As we have seen, five members of the Medicines Commission are chosen by ministers from the drug companies. Even worse, four members of the CSM have consultancies with pharmaceutical companies, a fact which the government was forced to admit after questions in Parliament. But the names and numbers of those with consultancies have only now made public (see page 98). The new committee which oversees the limited list (The Advisory Committee on NHS Drugs) is no different. Three of its members are drug company consultants and four own shares in drug companies. Furthermore, it can be safely assumed that almost all the clinicians on all the committees overseeing drug policy have worked, or will work on research projects sponsored by drug companies for which they, their junior researchers or their departmental colleagues will have received payment from the industry (see Chapter 2).

96

What effect do these close relationships have on the integrity and independence of the people chosen to regulate the drugs industry? Ultimately, that is a question for their own consciences. However, drug companies are very generous to those who serve them. A doctor who works on an *ad hoc* basis for a drug company – giving occasional advice and attending meetings irregularly – may receive only £1,000 a year. Those who are fully retained and advising regularly on company policy can expect to enjoy consultancy fees of at least £20,000 a year. Money talks, and it is hard for anyone to be truly impartial when it talks that loudly. There is nothing in law, however, to prevent these links. The pharmaceutical companies use sophisticated research and public relations techniques to identify all the influential clinicians who might one day be called upon to decide whether their drugs are suitable for sale. So great is the interweaving of interests that it is now virtually impossible to exclude experts who have links from sitting on the committees which regulate drugs. There are very few independent experts left.

The problem will not be solved simply by requiring an expert to declare his or her direct interests. If an expert is retained by company X, he or she will, conversely, have an interest in blocking the licensing of a rival drug made by company Y.

Dr Francis Roe is one of the members of the Committee on Toxicity at the Department of Health. As its name suggests, the COT has the solemn task of assessing whether permitted chemicals, be they drugs or food additives, are toxic and therefore too dangerous to use, regardless of their other benefits. Dr Roe was a paid consultant to the British Caramel Manufacturers Association at the very time (1986–87) when the COT was reassessing the safety of caramel colours (E150). Asked by the *Guardian* newspaper whether he felt any conflict of interest, Dr Roe said no, he did not. He had openly declared his consultancy, but the chairman of the COT, Professor Paul Turner, did not ask him to stand down from the debate.

Why did Dr Roe feel so free? He told the *Guardian* that he had so many consultancies, he did not feel purchased by any particular quarter. 'At any one time I am involved with

30-40 companies. I don't feel any need to defend one, to be truthful. I asked the chairman whether he wanted me to leave the room or not, but the fact is that on many occasions with the COT I would have to declare an interest on every item on the agenda.'[12] If not enough independent experts can be found to staff the sensitive health committees, then at the very least, all consultancies, links and ties should be declared quite publicly. The government moves at a snail's pace, and at last a pledge, made by Kenneth Clarke to the House of Commons in 1985 to come clean about links between the drug industry and the advisory committees has just been honoured. In October 1988 the 'personal interests' of the members of the Commission and of the various Section four committees were declared in their annual report.[13] Of the 24 Commission members 5 are full-time employees of the industry – the Medicines Act requires that at least one should have 'recent experience of the industry'. Of the remaining 19, several are listed as having 'personal interests' in drug companies, holding shares, consultancies and personally receiving fees. We are not told of the size of these 'personal' interests, nor whether the member holds a fellowship endowed by the industry, or receives grants from the industry for supporting staff or buying equipment. Were the professor of pharmacology of Oxford University an adviser, it seems possible that under the present arrangements he would not need to declare his interests, despite the fact that his department currently receives a grant of £5 million a year from Squibb.

Is there any evidence that this climate of secrecy allows poor medicines to be foisted on unsuspecting doctors and the public? The plain answer is, yes.

If only one thing mattered – the health of patients – then choosing good drugs would be easy. Before a new drug were allowed on the market proof would be needed that its combination of safety, efficacy and quality gave it advantages over any existing medicine for the same complaint or disease. If a new drug were only as good as existing therapies in these respects, it might still be licensed if it were cheaper to prescribe, easier to take, or both. These seem the kind of rules which any sensible government would adopt when drawing up legislation. But the Medicines Act falls far short of these straightforward tests. It does not allow the CSM to evaluate whether a new drug works as well (comparative efficacy) as existing therapies. If the new drug is deemed to be safe, and of consistent quality then it must be allowed for sale even if it does not work as well in treating disease as its established rivals. Moreover, the Act does not require the CSM to consider whether a new drug is cheaper or easier to take. So the Act provides no guide to cost, no guide to comparative efficacy, and no guide to ease of treatment. Since the law does not prevent the licensing of inferior drugs, and since licensing is done in secret by people with close links with the drug industry, is it any surprise that the nation's medicine chest includes many poor and unnecessarily expensive products?

Efficacy

The drug industry's bad behaviour might have been contained if the Medicines Act had at least provided a clear definition of drug *efficacy*: precise criteria by which the action of a drug against a specific disease or condition could be measured. If this sounds highly academic, it isn't. It is common sense. In medicine there can be five different responses when a drug is given to treat, say a rash.

First, the drug may ease the rash and nothing else happens. Second, it may ease the rash but also induce a harmful secondary response, for example, diarrhoea. The drug may only induce a harmless response, with no provable effect on the rash. Fourth, it may have no observable effect whatsoever, even though there is evidence from the laboratory that it should ease the rash. Finally, the drug may make the rash worse.

The only kind of efficacy that most people want from a drug is the first: that it works effectively to treat or cure a specific ailment, and does nothing else. The Medicines Act rules out drugs which produce only unwanted, harmful effects but it allows drugs with no proven therapeutic effect to be described as efficacious and to be marketed.

The law gives the benefit of doubt to the drug companies. It allows them to use flimsy extrapolations from animal studies, small healthy volunteer trials and even armchair postulation to justify their case for having their drug approved. Firm proof that the drug actually works among genuine patients suffering from the targeted complaint does not have to be provided. EEC regulations require[14] that all new drugs must provide clinical benefit and therapeutic effect in patients before they are licensed. But this sensible rule is ignored in Whitehall. So, unless a doctor is both knowledgeable and unsusceptible to drug company promotion, he is likely to prescribe any manner of inadequate but expensive remedies.

Allowing drugs with no therapeutic effect on to the market, wastes NHS and therefore taxpayers' money. It also threatens the lives of patients who may be denied access to a genuinely effective treatment because their doctors have been hoodwinked into prescribing medicines of unproven worth. The problem is not theoretical. In 1987 the drug Allpyral was withdrawn after years of use as 'therapy for patients known to suffer from grass pollen asthma'.[15] Specialists knew it offered little help in this condition; more to theepoint they knew it regularly killed people. Mianserin, a drug used for the last ten years for treating depression, poisons the bone marrow in about one in 10,000 patients, some of whom will die. Even now doctors question its effectiveness,[16] and when it was introduced the evidence was even weaker. The list goes on; impartial authorities have found no convincing evidence that Vasculit is effective for treating senile dementia,[17] that Opilon is effective for patients with poor circulation,[17] Persantin for strokes[18] or Stromba for leg ulcers.[19] When the limited list was introduced, hundreds of preparations were identified as essentially ineffective and withdrawn from NHS use overnight. But the *British National Formulary* still contains notes proclaiming 'there is no convincing evidence that drug X has a beneficial action'.

All these drugs have been licensed for years. Could it be that control has now become tighter? The straight answer, again, is no. In 1987 Faverin was introduced for the treatment of depression, but evidence for its claimed effects were unconvincing.[20] Stemetil Eff, Buccastem and Evoxin were introduced for the treatment of nausea and vomiting. Evidence for their claimed therapeutic efficacy is thin.[21, 22] In 1988 Buspar was launched. Trumpeted as a breakthrough in the treatment of anxiety, the *Lancet* noted, 'the drug is radical and new, but we will have to wait and see whether these qualities are therapeutic in anxiety'.[23]

The pharmaceutical industry likes to develop and license combination products – drugs with two or more allegedly active ingredients. It claims that patients benefit because they get the advantages of two or more drugs together. Combination drugs are often just marketing ploys – attempts to provide the illusion of novelty where none exists. The best selling antibiotic made by Wellcome is a combination product called Septrin. It is a mixture of two antimicrobial agents, trimethoprim and sulphamethoxazole. You might expect that ingredients combined in this way would do a useful job. And yet, when used to treat kidney and bladder infections (common enough complaints), Septrin is inappropriate because sulphamethoxazole provides no therapeutic advantage and may have serious disadvantages. Trimethroprim given alone treats these infections as effectively, and probably more safely.[24] Septrin's failings were never probed because drug authorities refuse to judge therapeutic efficacy in depth.

Under the Medicines Act, drug regulators should not be concerned with efficacy, a matter, the authorities argue, best left to doctors and their patients. Even if studies show that drug X is not as effective as drug Y, that is no reason to ban drug X from the market. Maybe drug X works better for some people, and doctors should have the freedom to choose. There is some merit to this argument. We know that the metabolism of individuals varies greatly and that different patients may react very differently to different drugs. Doctors should have the freedom to choose.

Is this what they are really getting? Very few doctors have the time, analytical skills or pharmacological knowledge to say, 'I know drug X is an outdated, expensive combination product which is unsuitable for most of my patients. By careful testing though, I have determined that it works brilliantly, for reasons I can't explain, on Mr So-and-So's sciatica.'

For every doctor who benefits from this freedom, hundreds drown in the quagmire of choice. With thousands of drugs to choose from, they can have no real idea what they all do –

which is exactly as the drug companies like it. So long as a doctor remains confused, he remains susceptible to the sales persuasion of drug company representatives. The government's assertive desire that it does not want to meddle in this market has nothing to do with the rights of doctors and patients, but concerns protecting the sales of the drug industry, which it is so keen to sponsor. This loyalty is most clearly exposed by looking for a moment at the doses of the medicines we are actually taking.

Dose: The Hidden Engine of Profit

Every manufacturer prays that their scientists will come up with a drug which is special. A drug with qualities that will distinguish it from all the other brands and give the promoters what they crave – a product with a 'unique selling point'. If there is nothing unique, which is generally the rule, the company will have to cook something up. Two classic selling points are 'greater effectiveness' and 'greater safety', and for marketing purposes each can be notionally achieved by manipulating the dose. A product made up at a high dose will certainly have greater effectiveness, and in some people this will be an advantage. It will also have more unwanted actions. Conversely, a product at a low dose is likely to be relatively free of side effects – and of course it will also have rather few wanted effects. This may sound silly but this is a balance that companies take most seriously. Knowing this, one might expect that the Department of Health would ensure that we only got as much of a drug as is really safe and necessary and yet the licensing authority fails even to consider the dose response of drugs, that is to say, the amount of a drug we need to get a desired therapeutic response. This failure has caused unnecessary deaths.

The heart drug captopril, whose discovery we discussed in chapter 1, was marketed at doses of up to 450 mg daily when it was first prescribed. How was this high dose for the treatment of high blood pressure arrived at? It is hard to say but we may assume that the licensing authority did not require the manufacturer, Squibb, to submit critical dose-response data when it applied for a licence. The flaw in the regulation led to tragic consequences. We now know that captopril's blood pressure lowering properties are fully at work once the patient is given a dose of no more than 150 mg a day, but at doses up to 450 mg captopril has been shown to damage the kidneys, and to depress production of blood cells in the bone marrow. Studies have shown that these potentially lethal side effects are most unlikely[25] to occur at lower doses.

Patients who were made ill or died from the effects caused by the high dosage did so unnecessarily. Moreover they suffered in silence – here was a 300% error in dose selection yet there was no public outcry and ministers and the manufacturer went unquestioned. Compare this to the response that followed the discovery that the radiotherapy department at the Royal Devon and Exeter Hospital had given a dose of treatment 25% above predicted.[26] Of course patients at Exeter were put at risk and it was right that a telephone hotline was established for the patients, that there were interviews with the press, and that experts, including the Health and Safety Executive, were called in. The contrast between Exeter and Whitehall is marked – the response to the licensing authority's mistake was a deafening silence.

The arthritis drug, Opren, is another case where high doses led to death. Many of the elderly people who died from taking Opren between 1980 and 1982 were poisoned because they took too much of the drug. The makers, it seems, chose to go for the upper end of the dose response curve for their product, and the DHSS accepted it apparently without question. Although the drug was potent at these doses it was also toxic. Those who got away with these high doses were grateful, those who didn't died. Elderly patients were particularly susceptible to the high doses. Had they been given smaller doses, they probably would have survived.

The number of drugs which the licensing authority allows to be sold in toxic doses is admittedly small. If enough people start dying, corrections, like the withdrawal of Opren and the reduction of the captopril dose, will begin to be made.

At least we know in these cases that a mistake has been made. Less dangerous, but more common are products which are made up in doses too small to be active. The aim is to create a feeling of security – never mind the fact it has no effect, at least it is safe. The drug Cetiprin was withdrawn in May 1988 after having been prescribed for over 20 years for urinary incontinence. It had just been 'discovered' that the drug was being used (and had been since its introduction) in doses too low to be effective. This is probably rather rare in drugs given singly, however it is almost always the case in combination products, where a manufacturer makes some claim about the 'synergistic' benefit of two or more active ingredients working together. It doesn't want to run the risk of causing unwanted effects so it uses only a minute amount of one of the ingredients. After all, nobody will check, and the manufacturer has made himself a product that is unique.

A good example of a popular drug with an ineffective ingredient is the combination product Migraleve, a treatment which is sold for the relief of migraine headaches. The makers of Migraleve make much in their advertisements of the need to take the different strength pink and yellow tablets at different stages of an attack. Yet one of the ingredients, buclizine, is probably never present at a strength which would be clinically effective and capable of justifying the manufacturer's claims that it helps bring relief to migraine sufferers.

The dose of a drug is, in any event, a pretty crude indicator of its real strength in combatting disease. What really matters is how much of the drug is absorbed into the blood stream and the effect this produces. Dose is just one factor. The way a drug is presented (tablet or capsule for instance) and the innate metabolism of each patient will also affect levels reached in the blood.

The licensing authority, however, often ignores absorption for generic products. For some, like the anti-epilepsy drug, phenytoin, and the heart drug, digoxin, the CSM will want to know how much of the drug reaches the blood after the tablet is taken and a licence will only be given if the figures match the market leader. However for many generics this seems not to be done.

Take a drug like the hypnotic temazepam, probably the most commonly prescribed 'sleeper' in the UK. Temazepam is marketed by several drug companies in 10 and 20mg capsules, and for each strength it was natural to regard the generic alternatives as interchangeable. This, however, is untrue; the capsules come in either a soft or a hard form and after being swallowed the soft form releases its contents much more quickly.[27] Unbeknown to doctors (and presumably the CSM) patients taking the hard capsule were taking longer to fall asleep and longer to recover. Come the morning this could become crucial for many people. Emotionally, the extra hour's blood levels may make them unable to function with their families over breakfast. Worse, they may then drive to work with coordination and concentration impaired, as if they were over the alcohol limit.

The whole issue of dose and absorption lies at the centre of the argument over generic prescribing. Can we be certain that the cheaper, generic alternative is absorbed identically to the famous, more expensive branded product. Since the licensing authority requires so little testing, it is hard to answer that question. From my experience, important differences in therapeutic efficacy between generic and branded drugs are rare. Nevertheless, the authority's complacency allows doubt to be sown. Doctors know that the cheaper generic will be made to the same dose as the branded drug they are familiar with. But they will have no proof, as they should have, that its absorption rate is identical. Moreover, as we will see later, there is indirect evidence that they can indeed differ. This uncertainty gives the big drug companies the opportunity they want to convince doctors to remain loyal to their expensive brands.

In the United States the Food and Drug Administration requires that the 'manufacturer of a generic drug must demonstrate that its product's rate and extent of absorption do not differ from those of the brand name product on which the initial approval was based'.[28] If this commonsense rule were applied in the UK, then many of the genuine concerns about generic substitution could be allayed. The authorities have no desire, however, to provide patients with the best possible drugs at the cheapest prices. Generic cost-cutting would doubtless reduce the financial pressure on the National Health Service while actually improving the medicines prescribed to patients. The pharmaceutical lobby would not like it.

Adverse Drug Reactions: Preventing the Next Thalidomide or Opren from Reaching the Market

At least all of us – doctors, consumers and pharmaceutical companies – are agreed that dangerous drugs should be withdrawn from the market. But how, exactly, should safety be measured? Does a chemical treatment for a terminal cancer need to be as safe as tablets to relieve cold symptoms? Ultimately, it is the job of the CSM to decide when drugs are too dangerous to use. The CSM has a positive obligation to assess the comparative safety of one drug against another. At first it relies on the data provided solely by the company, but after marketing it can use independent information. Opren might have stayed on the market (with an extra hazard warning) if it had been the only available drug of its kind to treat the pain of arthritis. Individual patients are not really part of the equation. The Medicines Act is concerned only with the health of the community (Section 132:2, (a)). Ultimately, the CSM is not principally interested, therefore, in the intrinsic safety of any given drug. Rather, it seeks to compare its risks to the dangers of the disease it is combating and to the risk profile of any alternative therapies.

There is usually disagreement, however, on whether the evidence justifies banning a suspected drug from the market. A doctor who thinks the drug is ineffective will be delighted to see it go, but the pharmaceutical company which has invested millions in its development and waited years to have it approved, may lobby ferociously to keep it on the market, arguing that its proven benefits easily outweigh its alleged dangers. Genuine differences of opinion will rage because accurately spotting adverse drug reactions (ADRs) is not easy. For example, most of the more common adverse effects such as headache, diarrhoea, indigestion, dizziness, itch, rash, impotence and general feeling of weakness occur just as often, with equal intensity, in people who, as part of the control group in an experiment, receive a placebo 'drug' which ought to have no effect on them whatsoever.

Some ADRs, though, are unequivocal. Normally sighted people who take the heart drug, digoxin, may begin to see things tinged with yellow, as though through yellow-tinted spectacles. This effect is never mentioned by patients on placebo. One can also say, with some certainty, that antibiotics cause diarrhoea, because the frequency of diarrhoea in people taking antibiotics is so great that there can be no doubt about the causal link between the two. There is also the provable, albeit rare, link between antibiotics and catastrophic diarrhoea with bleeding, which is life-threatening.

It may still, however, take decades to prove a link between a particular drug and a dangerous adverse reaction. This is because the reaction will occur in only a tiny proportion of patients. Most thalidomide and Opren patients took the drug and survived without any adverse 'reactions' whatsoever. And, as we have seen, most of the conditions that present as adverse reactions are occurring already, in the normal population, for no particular reason. It is extremely difficult, therefore, to prove that drug X caused reaction Y when most people who take drug X experience *no* adverse reaction, and when some sufferers of reaction Y have never taken drug X.

The dilemma was recently illustrated in the High Court (March 1988) when the parent of an alleged whooping cough vaccine victim failed to prove any causal link between the vaccine, subsequent fits and permanent brain damage. It has been widely assumed for years that the vaccine can cause severe reactions in up to one in 100,000 recipients. The judge ruled that there was insufficient evidence to establish that the vaccine had caused brain damage in the particular case.

Even when an adverse reaction is identified and proven, someone still has to decide whether it should be tolerated. For example, the authority would not permit major reactions to any drug used for a mild condition, such as a cold. At the other extreme, even severe adverse reactions may be acceptable if the drug is likely to save or at least prolong life. Many of the drugs used in chemotherapy to treat cancer are highly toxic. So too is AZT, or Retrovir, the AIDS drug made by Wellcome which stops the HIV virus from replicating, but which is also destructive to bone marrow, and can cause nerve damage, diarrhoea and muscle pains.

Some adverse reactions are frequent, severe and prolonged, but are tolerated because the alternative – no effective treatment – is worse. For example, corticosteroids will with few exceptions relieve even the most severe forms of asthma. The penalty for such life–saving treatment, however, is a swollen face, acne, unwanted hairiness (hirsutism), general weakness, the risk of developing diabetes, high blood pressure and even fragile bones. Corticosteroid use in asthma is permitted, however, because there is no safer alternative. In fact, a doctor who declines to give corticosteroids to severe asthma sufferers might be considered negligent, and in my experience, asthmatics rarely refuse this treatment. Tragically, one of my patients did refuse and she died unnecessarily at the age of 31, leaving behind a devoted husband and a four-year-old son.

Danger Signals

When it comes to spotting rogue drugs, the CSM has been one of the most successful worldwide,[29] even though the evidence from which it works is relatively sparse.

When a company applies for a product licence for a new drug, it is required by the CSM to list all the untoward reactions, whether directly attributable or merely suspected, experienced by patients during the drug's development. Typically, though, a new drug will have been tested in no more than 3,000 patients. This is too few, statistically, to spot all but the most conspicuous or frequent adverse reactions. A drug producing rapid elongation of the nose would quickly come to light. But if a new drug causes, say, severe anaemia, in one in every 50,000 patients, the reaction may never even occur in a single patient during the drug's development, and, in any case, anaemia may have many causes. Proving a causal link between the drug and the effect would be very difficult in this case.

Once a drug is on the market, its potential as a killer is still likely to go undetected. A typical GP prescribing the drug throughout his lifetime may never see a single adverse reaction, yet, if the drug is popular and widely used over many years, an ADR incidence of one in 50,000 will eventually bring a death toll of horrendous proportions. This is exactly what happened with the butazones, a group of powerful painkillers discovered and heavily marketed by the Swiss firm, Ciba Geigy.

Although the butazones were very effective painkillers, they also caused bone marrow depression which led to anaemia, bleeding and increased susceptibility to infection in about one in 50,000 people who were prescribed the drugs for more than one month. Between 1964, when they were first marketed, and 1985 it is estimated that the butazones were responsible for killing 1,000 people in the UK.[30]

Ciba Geigy continued strenuously to defend the safety of its drug and to dismiss any correlation between its use and these adverse reactions. But the CSM, under pressure from doctors and consumer groups, finally banned all uses of the butazones with the exception of a rare, debilitating and painful form of arthritis. The signal, pointing to the toll of death, had finally become distinct over a number of years and widespread use of the drugs simply could not be justified any longer.

Warning Beacons

The Committee on the Safety of Medicines sits in the dark. It needs eyes and ears to spot drug dangers. Information comes from the medical journals, where doctors' early concerns are raised; from the use of the yellow card system; by use of the 'prescription event monitoring' system, and finally, from information which pharmaceutical companies are supposed to report when they suspect their own drugs of causing adverse reactions.

The medical journals have proved most useful in the past. The problems of thalidomide were first exposed through letters written by doctors.[31] Similarly, the horrible reactions which patients suffered to ICI's second-generation heart drug, Eraldin, first came to light in the medical journals. More recently too, early warnings about the hazards of Opren in the elderly were reported by one doctor who was concerned that six of his patients had died while on the arthritis drug.

Journals are a fine thing – for those doctors with enough self-confidence and time to submit articles, but for most doctors, sending a letter or an article to the *Lancet* is a daunting prospect. For them a quick way of sending a warning message is crucial. It is called the yellow card. Almost every doctor is familiar with it. A few yellow cards are bound into the back of the *British National Formulary* and to prescription pads. They enable doctors who think they have seen an adverse reaction in a patient to make a quick note of the symptoms and suspected cause. The card is then sent away to the Department of Health for instant analysis.

That is the theory, anyway. The yellow card system was first introduced in 1964 and during its early years less than 3,500 a year were sent in by doctors to the Department of Health.[32] By 1986 the figure had climbed to 15,527.[33] This seems a good improvement, and statistically it is, but there are 24,000 GPs in the UK, so on average they are sending in less than one yellow card per year. The true picture is actually much worse. Yellow cards, are used by only a minority of doctors. It has been estimated that 90% of all the yellow cards are submitted by just 10% of all GPs. And in recent years a quarter of all yellow card reports sent in by doctors have focused on one single class of drugs – the non steroidal anti-inflammatory drugs (NSAIDs) used to control arthritis pain. This upsurge in reporting undoubtedly reflects all the attention that has rightly been given to the dangers of Opren, Surgam, Feldene and other drugs in the class. But it also means, comparatively, that GPs have been even more neglectful about sending in reports on other drugs.

The CSM has tried to pinpoint better reporting by asking doctors to be extra vigilant when prescribing new drugs – all of which are now denoted by a black triangle next to their entry in the *British National Formulary*. Any reaction seen in a patient, no matter how trivial or minor should be reported if it might be linked with the new drug.

Professor Bill Inman, who directs the Drug Safety Research Unit at the University of Southampton, has made adverse drug reactions his life's work.[34] He believes GPs fail spontaneously to send in yellow cards for a mixture of reasons. They fear litigation and ridicule if a subsequent investigation suggests that the adverse reaction was caused because they prescribed an inappropriate drug. Other GPs complacently believe that the authorities already know about any problem they might have spotted, or they doubt their own ability to distinguish between a true reaction to a drug and an unconnected event. Worst of all, a minority of doctors withhold reports and keep their suspicions secret in hopes of later winning fame by publishing their concerns in journals! What is needed, of course, is a way of spotting adverse reactions the moment they occur, and then networking them so that they all arrive at CSM.

Such a method, in its infancy, already exists, and it too was devised by Professor Inman. After a medicine is dispensed the chemist sends the original prescription to the Prescription Pricing Authority (PPA) using it as a claim for reimbursement. But they can be used for more than reimbursement. By inspecting the scripts the PPA can also discover which patient has received what and when. Working in conjunction with Professor Inman, scripts for selected drugs are earmarked and the prescribing doctors are sent letters asking how their patients have fared.

The system seems foolproof. All patients who have received a drug over a set period are identified and their health monitored-prescription event monitoring (PEM). However, the system has had some serious shortcomings in that it failed to detect that troublesome effects of Opren, and more recently missed Mianserin's effect on the blood (see page 100). At present the verdict on the PEM system must be 'value unproven'.

The most direct method of tracing unwanted effects is by making use of computers used in doctors' surgeries to log case notes and prescriptions. Unfortunately, the Department of Health has refused to help to fund or organize a national computer system for doctors which would be safe from prying eyes. Instead, at least two private firms are now competing in this highly sensitive, but also potentially lucrative market. They are offering doctors free computers in return for their prescribing data. What is the catch? It is that the computer firms make their money by selling the prescribing data back to the pharmaceutical industry. The prime interest which the drug companies have in these data is not their desire to catch their own drugs going wrong, although there is an element of this. Their principal motive is marketing, not good medicine.

They want to see how well their drugs are performing against rival brands. This kind of marketing information is gleaned all the time by makers of chocolate bars and soap powders who then use it to redefine and redirect their advertising and sales promotion campaigns. The selling of prescription drugs and soap powder have always been very different for the simple reason that people only need drugs when they are ill, and when they are, their doctors should not be under promotional pressure to switch brands.

The fear is that if the drug companies can buy computer data from doctors, then doctors will become even less vigilant in reporting adverse reactions to the authorities. This might not be so bad, if the drug companies could be trusted to regulate themselves. In theory, they are required, as part of the provisions of the product licence they hold, to report to the CSM any adverse reactions that they spot in their products. They have special company yellow forms[35] for doing so.

They are also pressed (although there is no legal requirement) to seek out adverse reactions when they design post-marketing surveillance trials. Unfortunately, as we have seen in chapter 2, drug companies have used these trials as cynical marketing ploys to boost their share. Bayer, the West German drugs giant, offered gifts and cash payments to British doctors in bogus trials designed merely to switch more patients on to its brand of heart drug, Adalat. The industry claims that these trials are done in search of further evidence of a product's efficacy, for improvements in the dosage regimen or for indications that it may be useful in a new therapeutic area. It also claims that the studies may be undertaken specifically to collect adverse reaction data. In the case of Bayer's study, however, the forms which doctors filled out were never even sent back to the company's headquarters.

The Failure Within Whitehall

Let us imagine that all drug companies could suddenly be persuaded to put patient health before profit and all doctors became vigilant in reporting adverse reactions. If all this accurate and unbiased information poured into the Department of Health, what would happen? Probably, an almighty snarl-up. The government commissioned a report into the workings of the Medicines Division in 1987.[36] It found that the division was hopelessly inadequate and under-funded. The limited computer system was ancient, and many important files were, or so it seems, untraceable.

It may seem odd that the government should commission such a report. It has, after all, a duty under the Medicines Act to regulate drugs effectively. Why then, should it choose to publish a report which so glaringly admits that morale at the Medicines Division is low, its equipment is antediluvian, and its personnel not of the highest calibre?

The answer, perhaps, is that the government is looking for a backdoor way of privatising the Medicines Division. The authors of the report (John Evans and Peter Cunliffe) suggested that the pharmaceutical companies be brought in to pay completely for the regulatory service. They also suggested that the industry should play a prominent part in the budget committee that would influence how staff are chosen, and how much they would be paid. The idea that Britain should have a strong and independent drugs regulatory agency (like the US Food and Drug Administration) is not even seriously considered. Perhaps the conclusions that the report reached should be obvious given that one of the authors, Peter Cunliffe, was the former managing director of ICI Pharmaceuticals division.

At every turn, the Medicines Division shows itself reluctant to get tough with the drug companies. EEC legislation actually requires it to judge the comparative efficacy of rival drugs. It states that for all licensed drugs 'therapeutic advantage must outweigh clinical risk'.[14] Ministers would no doubt claim that the CSM does adhere to all European requirements, but this is palpably untrue; drugs continue to be licensed and re-licensed (see below) when their clinical efficacy has not been seriously assessed and they have not been fairly compared with rival drugs.

If the Medicines Division had the slightest desire to get tough with drug companies, then it would use power of licence renewal to remove older drugs as better ones become available. All drugs must be relicensed every five years. Ideally, their comparative efficacy and safety should be examined. In practice, this seldom happens. As a result, some patients are denied improved therapy while others have been injured or even killed by lethal drugs left unreasonably on the market.

In theory an old drug must be withdrawn if it is superseded by a genuinely better and safer alternative. What is never made public is how large this 'health gap' needs to be before the authorities take action. In practice, the withdrawal of a licence is very rare and the initiative to cease marketing is usually left to the manufacturer. Lack of initiative is a hallmark of the division. It responds to industry, or occasionally to critics, rather than taking the lead. It seems to do little even when ample evidence exists that change would improve patient welfare.

It has been known for several years that about a quarter of available drugs are made of molecules that can exist in two forms, one a mirror image of the other. Of the two forms, only one is therapeutically active; the other is an impurity that can cause unwanted effects. By changing the synthetic process, all these drugs could be produced in pure form, but the Division has never dared to insist that this should be done. Rather than confronting the manufacturers and demanding, for instance, that they should produce only the beneficial form of ethambutol because the impurity causes blindness, the companies were left to do as they please. And the position remains the same today.

Perhaps the CSM feels this would be too great a confrontation, but it avoids even the smallest of challenges. Steroid tablets used in asthma and other inflammatory conditions have the most unpleasant side effects, but over the years ways have been devised to reduce them. If a drug like prednisolone is given on alternate days, and then only as a single dose in the early morning, many of the problems are avoided – children will not be stunted, neither will diabetes develop, etc. This has been recognized since at least 1976,[37] but the advice in the data sheets still makes no mention of this regimen. Manufacturers are still recommending that steroids should be taken every day, throughout the day. The CSM should have ensured that the manufacturers' instructions were changed.

Even when drugs are measured for their consistent and uniform quality the authorities are lenient toward the industry. Measuring the purity, sterility and stability of a compound ought to be quite uncontroversial. Moreover, it is important that generic equivalents of branded formulations do contain identical ingredients which break down in the same way to give the same concentration in the body, and the alleged quality of a drug may have a real impact on its performance. Many tablets and capsules claim to have a mechanism to speed, slow or target the release of the medicine. For example, a new formulation of salicylic acid called Asacol, which is for the treatment of ulcerative colitis, claims a special coating that targets the release of the medicine to the large intestine, the part of the digestive system affected by these conditions. Scientists in the Medicines Division are responsible for assessing whether these claims of quality are met consistently. A recent study showed, however, that quality control of UK drugs is woefully unreliable. When three thousand random analyses were performed on medicines by Regional Quality Controllers in 1987, 29% revealed defects and failure to reach specification.[38] Some of the flaws were trivial, but not all. Tests conducted on the anti-epileptic drug, phenobarbitone, were particularly alarming. They showed that some tablets of the drug dissolved completely within five minutes of being added to the test system, while others took more than an hour.

A spokeswomen from the Medicines Division denied that such differences were real and suggested they reflected poor analytical techniques. In the Division's hands, she said, quality controls on generics always showed the products to be identical. This confidence is not shared by the hospital service, whose regions employ quality control pharmacists who routinely check generic alternatives before they allow them to be used.

It is also quite wrong that drug manufacturers should face less stringent requirements on ingredient labelling than food manufacturers. The makers of *Smarties* must list which colours they use to coat their famous sweets. By contrast drug manufacturers who use tartrazine (E102), the controversial yellow colorant, are still under no obligation to disclose this, even though tartrazine can cause severe allergic reactions in some people. Patients who are already severely ill may be

115

unable to withstand the further stress of an intolerance reaction to the colorant.

There are moves afoot to change these arrangements and by the summer of 1989 the DHSS plans, at long last, to list in the data sheet and other leaflets for doctors or pharmacists all of a product's inactive ingredients.[39] There may, however, be some delay since the industry will be arguing that disclosure should not be total,[40] and consumer groups will argue that the information should also be available to patients.

Perhaps the most disconcerting evidence on the Medicines Division comes from the Faverin affair; not because the drug itself is particularly dangerous, but because of the incompetence exposed in the section of the Division that deals with the yellow card system – a system seen as the jewel in the Authority's crown. In May 1988 the CSM reported in the *British Medical Journal*[41] that since 1986 there had been five suspected deaths due to the antidepressant drug Faverin. In June 1988 the *Observer* newspaper reported this accurately after receiving a circular from the DHSS which gave the same figure as had appeared in the *BMJ*.[42] Within days of the publication of the *Observer* article, a spokesperson from the Medicines Division told me, and rather sternly at that, that the deaths were not an effect of the drug, but rather a 'chance association', an about turn later repeated in a DHSS press release.[43] Such muddles seem to confirm the findings in the Evans-Cunliffe inquiry of a government department underfunded and with staff calibre well below par.

Walls of Secrecy

There is only one explanation for the unfairness, inconsistency and inefficiencies of British drugs policy: it is formulated and conducted by a closed band of ministers and civil servants who choose to consult only the pharmaceutical industry before making public decisions in private. Even doctors have no right to information. Section 118 of the Medicines Act enshrines secrecy as the legal method of our masters' conduct. It is even forbidden for any member of the Medicines Division to divulge to a doctor the names of the ingredients in any drug formulation. We, as patients and citizens, have no right to know why a drug was approved for sale, on what grounds it was considered safe and effective, and what exactly each medicine contains.

Even the work of the Medicines Commission itself is secret. Its advice to ministers in the Department of Health remains confidential, and its annual report contains only details of the Commission's constitution and membership, and a few paragraphs summarizing its achievements. For example, when appeals against suspension of drug licences are discussed, there is no mention of the name of the drug, the issues surrounding its withdrawal, or the manufacturer. Yet the Medicines Commission is supposed to be the independent body which guarantees that the public gets the top quality medical treatment it deserves. Instead, it has been reduced to a small cog in the secret machine of the national stealth, designed to maintain a quiet life for civil servants and ministers and ample profits for the drug companies. It no longer has any real authority. It was not formally consulted when the government decided to establish the limited list. It played no visible role when the government chose to evaluate the cost and effectiveness of the drug regulators within the Medicines Division.[36]

If doctors were regularly consulted, or at least had the right to ask questions, then it is likely that some of the more dangerous, but merely derivative, anti-arthritis drugs would never have got on the market. They would have been able to say, 'Look, we already have enough of these drugs. They all relieve pain to some extent, but they all have serious side effects. Don't confuse us with another one until it genuinely provides a higher level of pain relief, or it is genuinely kinder to the stomach, kidneys and liver.'

Instead, the drug companies are able to submit applications for endless variants of old drugs. Often, as the Medicines Commission[44] and the Evans and Cunliffe inquiry have both complained, drug company applications are inadequate and incomplete. It would be instructive to see what kind of drug applications the companies might submit if confidentiality were lifted. Would they be cajoled into submitting well-documented applications, for only those drugs with genuine new properties?

In the United States the Food and Drug Administration is required to publish a Summary Statement of Approval which explains in outline why a new product has been given a licence. Since the FDA has to summarize the data anyway, it was assumed that its publication might be helpful to the public. When requests were made in Britain for similar publication of drug data, the suggestion was dismissed as being 'uneconomical'. It was suggested that all necessary information could be obtained through questions in the House of Commons[36] – a very slow process.

The Medicines Division is also prevented from a full and frank exchange of information with the equivalent regulatory agencies in other countries. By contrast, the USA and Scandinavian countries regularly circulate reports of their meetings which detail why drug licences were granted. The Australians go even further, sending out circulars which explain why they have refused permission for a new drug to be marketed. Ironically it almost looked as though the CSM would be trapped by its own secrecy. For years the authority has been comparing information in one licence with that in another. It is, in fact, no more than common sense to assess a new product by comparing it with an earlier one. But if the contents of the original application are secret how can they be referred to when considering a second application? This principle formed the basis of a case brought against the DHSS by the American multinational Smith, Kline and French (SK&F). As a result, from December 1987 till the summer of 1988 the CSM was barred from using data which SK&F supplied when assessing applications from other companies.[45] The processing of applications to market copies of SK&F's drug Tagamet was at a standstill. Fortunately for the CSM, SKF's case was lost on appeal and Section 119 remains intact.[46]

Profits

Drug companies declare how much profit they make in the United States, but they refuse, almost without exception, ever to state publicly how much profit they earn in Britain from the National Health Service. Nor do they have to: their profits, earned from national insurance contributors, and set by Whitehall civil servants are, in effect, a national secret.

Each year, each drug company is told how many millions it will make from the NHS. Competition does not exist for the pharmaceutical industry. Instead, profits are allocated in secret under the Pharmaceuticals Price Regulation Scheme, or PPRS for short. The deal is so cosy that it is worth explaining it in some detail.

Let's invent a fictional drug company, Collier plc. It makes a range of heart drugs, anti-arthritis pain killers and inhalers for asthma. Once a year Collier plc goes along to the Department of Health and states how much capital (money) it is employing in making drugs which the NHS buys. Let us say that it is £100 million, or so Collier plc claims. Collier plc is also asked how much it is spending on promoting its drugs to doctors and how much it is spending on research and development.

If Collier plc is clever, it will claim that its post market surveillance trials (in reality promotional gimmicks designed to boost sales of its products) are really research tools designed to help it find new adverse reactions to its drugs. Collier plc will claim this because the government will penalize it for doing too much promotion, but reward it for doing research and development.

The Department of Health will then decide that Collier plc deserves a 25% return on its capital employed. This means, since it claims to have invested £100 million, that it is entitled to earn a £25 million profit from the NHS. To collect its profits, Collier then sets what prices it likes on its drugs, based on the likely number of tablets and injectables it is likely to sell.

In the early 1980s the government chose to tighten the formula, and the drug companies complained that they were only earning profits in the target range of 16–21%. But the rules have been relaxed in recent years, and companies which invest heavily in research and show good export records can now expect to earn profits of up to 30% a year from the NHS.

Even this kind of figure is likely to be an underestimate of the true earnings of drug companies. By pretending to charge themselves a lot for cheap chemicals imported from foreign subsidiaries (a practice known as transfer pricing), the companies can artificially inflate the capital employed and thereby disguise the true profits they are making. The government promised several years ago to investigate transfer pricing. But its findings, if any, were never made public.

Promotion

The government has abdicated virtually all responsibility for controlling how drug companies promote their products. Only once (see Chapter 2) has a major company been prosecuted for bogus advertising. Policing is left mainly to the code of practice committee run by the Association of the British Pharmaceutical Industry. Its sessions are confidential. A company may have committed all manner of sins in falsely promoting its product. It may have taken doctors and their partners on lavish foreign trips, and grossly exaggerated claims for the drugs in advertisements. But the ABPI's code of practice committee will censure with the utmost discretion, publishing only a brief and blandly worded adjudication.

These excesses would be less abhorrent if, at least, the Medicines Division made a real effort to force the drug companies to produce absolutely accurate and up-to-the-minute data sheets on their drugs. Their sheets are controlled by law and should contain only information that has been approved by the Authority. Strict control though is hardly the rule.

A good example of the Medicine Division's laggardly approach is the data sheet on the drug Persantin (dipyridamole) produced by the German firm, Boehringer Ingleheim. It claimed that the drug should be used to treat strokes and heart attacks and 'diseases or conditions where modification of platelet function may be beneficial', that is, conditions where blood clots are likely. There is, in fact, not one shred of convincing clinical evidence to support this claim.[47] Yet on three successive occasions the Medicines Division renewed the data sheet for Persantin without any apparent criticism. It was only revised after a blistering attack was made in the *Drug and Therapeutics Bulletin*.[18]

This failure is not an isolated example. In 1983 the

Committee on the Safety of Medicines advised that all data sheets for products likely to be used by the elderly should, by 1985, contain particular prescribing advice for older people. The advice followed the withdrawal of Opren in 1982. The CSM wanted the dangers of gastro-intestinal bleeding and perforation to be spelt out for this class of drug. But the warnings of the CSM were blatantly ignored and the data sheet for the market leader Feldene (piroxicam) remained unchanged by the end of 1985.

The CSM was hardly asking the drug companies to address themselves to some arcane point of pharmacology. It was simply saying that the elderly needed to be protected from the misuse of the kind of drugs which had been proven to be dangerous to them. Early in 1986 the CSM published more data stressing the gastrointestinal dangers to the elderly.[48] It warned doctors that 'in the elderly these drugs should be given only after other forms of treatment have been carefully considered', and that 'it is prudent to start treatment at the bottom end of the dose range'.

The response from the industry, however, was begrudging and minimal. Most companies chose to make only obscure reference to the problem and one firm, Thomas Morson, part of MSD, blatantly ignored the CSM's advice by continuing to state for its drug, Dolobid, that 'the dosage does not require modification for elderly patients'.

There is no excuse for out-of-date sheets, and considering the criticism they have received one might have expected the Medicines Division to be more vigilant. But in 1987 data sheets were still being published that were hopelessly out-of-date. There was, for instance, no mention of drug dependence in the sheets for three benzodiazepine drugs, and a statement that the local anaesthetic ointment 'Xyloproct' had no 'known contraindications or side effects' is wrong.[49]

Particularly noteworthy in 1988 was the data sheet for the Transiderm Nitro skin patches. For years researchers had argued that this preparation lost its effect as a treatment for angina when used continuously.[50] If it was to remain effective it should be applied intermittently and perhaps for only 14 hours in every 24.[51] Despite this information the data sheet has continued to advise that the patch be applied continuously day in, day out – a regimen that almost certainly renders the product ineffective within days or weeks.

The Medicines Act clearly stipulates that advertisements should be consistent with the data sheet, the data sheet consistent with the licence and the licence consistent with verifiable evidence. It is also the positive duty of Health Ministers to enforce the act (Section 180, 1) and they could be brought before a judicial review for failing in that duty.

If the government genuinely wished to control the promotional excesses of the drug industry, it would set up a new section 4 committee, perhaps called the Committee on the Promotion of Medicines (CPM) which would rank in authority along side the CSM. Doctors who were worried about advertisements and data sheets would then have a court of direct appeal rather than being forced, as now, to express their misgivings to the drug industry's own code of practice committee.

A new committee on the promotion of medicines should also press for changes in the Medicines Act to allow comparative assessment of drugs on data sheets. Doctors would then, for example, be able to see at a glance whether the drug was more or less likely than another to cause gastrointestinal bleeding in the elderly.

Unfortunately, the government shows no inclination to make drug policy more accessible and accountable. Even when it did a good thing – establishing the limited list – it did so for the wrong reason (a desire merely to save money), and it again cloaked the whole business in secrecy.

The Advisory Committee on Drugs (ACD), which was set up in June 1985 to run the limited list, was established in such haste that its existence was neither approved by parliament nor is its role governed by any legislation. It owes its existence merely to a statement in the House of Commons made by the Secretary of State for Social Services.[52] It operates in obscurity. Its members were all asked to abide by the Official Secrets Act, and it publishes no report of its activities. It is answerable to no one except the Minister. Applications to add new drugs to the list are supposed to take 3–4 months, but delays of up to 18 months occur. The limited list also falsely claims to meet 'all clinical needs', which is nonsense.

When first drafted in November 1984 the limited list excluded many useful drugs merely on the grounds of cost. Obviously, if five drugs with indistinguishable properties exist, then the cheapest and the cheapest alone should be chosen. But safety, efficacy and convenience of usage are all more important than cost. Fortunately, the limited list was so altered during the consultation period that it came finally to resemble very closely a list produced by the Drugs and Therapeutics Bulletin and based on the views of almost one hundred leading UK clinicians who were asked to select medicines on health, rather than cost, grounds. Nevertheless, the DHSS saved £75 million in the first year of operation.[53] Saving money can be easily compatible with patient welfare.

Public Parsimony: Cancer Screening

The government is still largely failing to control drug industry profits, but at the same time it refuses to spend prudently to improve preventive medicine – a step which would not only save suffering and lives but, in the long term, hard cash as well. It is as if the government only understands the value of balancing the NHS books, while having no grasp whatsoever of the true value of health.

This paucity of vision and parsimony of purse is nowhere more evident than in the government's dishonest failure to set up adequate cervical and breast screening programmes for women. Around 2,000 women die in England and Wales each year from cervical cancer. The death toll could be halved if we had an adequate screening programme.[54] This discovery is hardly new. It has been known since the late 1960s, from worldwide information, that deaths from cervical cancer could be greatly reduced if women had a systematic programme for collecting and analysing cervical smears – sample cells scraped from the neck of the uterus. All women in 'at risk' categories above an agreed age should be recalled for a smear test every three years until they reach 65. Since it takes several years for the microscopic changes in the cells to become truly cancerous, screening ought to save almost every woman from this preventable death.

In the early 1980s the government asked the Committee for

Gynaecological Cytology to review cervical cancer treatment in Britain. The committee issued two reports (1981, 1984), both strongly urging that national guidelines be set up, to allow every local authority to contribute to a national computerized system for calling and recalling every woman in the country in 'at risk' categories for cervical screening. The committee also called for a nationwide publicity campaign to heighten public awareness.

The government's response was, however, largely negative. It decided there should be no publicity campaign. Arrangements for a centralized computer were scrapped. No attempt was made to coordinate a national programme and no money was given to support local initiatives.

More damning evidence was to emerge in 1985. A survey[54] showed that one third of all district health authorities had no cervical screening programme whatsoever. Of those programmes that did exist, a quarter were manually operated and therefore lacked any reliable way to track and contact women in the scheme. Only three percent of the districts had call-and-recall schemes similar to those recommended. Even when screening was available, results were handled erratically. By 1987 it was still often taking three months to relay results of a smear test to the referring doctor, even though the few better-run districts were proving that replies could be sent to doctors within a fortnight.[55] In many instances positive results (indicating early cancer) would never have been reported to the patient,[56] some of whom will have died.

In the face of these terrible statistics, the government's bravado was chilling. The Department of Health's official review of health statistics boasted in 1987 that, 'there has been a gradual decline in the number of deaths from cervical cancer although there was a slight rise between 1982 and 1983 and again between 1984 and 1985.'

The Secretary of State for Social Services assured us that just over half of the health districts of England and Wales would have full screening systems by the end of March 1987. But this claim was revealed to be a gross exaggeration. A survey by Frank Dobson,[54] the then shadow Health Minister, revealed that only 21 of the 75 districts cited by the Secretary of State actually had call-and-recall screening. And only eight of the districts had adopted the most meticulous standards (women over 20 screened every three years) advocated by many experts in the field. True to form, government ministers denied the accusations, claiming the screening programme was on schedule and that the opposition had got it wrong. But the criticism did not go away.

By early 1988 the Committee of the Medical Royal Colleges[57] and Harriet Harman,[58] the shadow Minister of Health, both reported studies showing that cervical screening remained woefully inadequate. The government had promised a fully operational national scheme by April 1 1988 but these reports found that in only two thirds of the UK was the service ready.

The death rate in the UK from cervical cancer has fallen slightly since 1981, but it is still much higher than in countries of comparable affluence and medical sophistication. Nine out of ten women who die will not have been tested,[57] and that is the outcome of government policy. Why don't the experts complain? They can't do so. As government advisers, which many are, they will have signed the Official Secrets Act.

The government's record in preventing breast cancer is just as poor. Breast cancer kills about 5,000 women each year in the UK between the ages of 50 and 65. The death toll could be reduced by over a third if screening programmes like those in Sweden and the United States were adopted. The Forrest Committee was asked by government for its views and it recommended that for all women between the ages of 50 and 64 there should be a call-and-recall screening programme.[59] Such a national system would need 120 screening units and would cost £31 million to set up and another £18 million each year to run.

The government accepted the Forrest Committee recommendations and said it was moving swiftly to implement them.[60] Then at a press conference the government said it would make available £6 million to launch a breast screening programme in 14 units,[61] somewhat short of the £31 million suggested by Forrest. The government clearly thought it could get £49 million worth of publicity for £6 million and that it could establish 14 breast screening units when its own expert committee recommended 120. The committee, like all others, had been sworn to secrecy.

This attitude toward two of the biggest killers of women contrasts oddly with the government's recent prevention programme against AIDS, a disease which, so far, has largely affected males. No one would deny that the £20 million educational campaign against AIDS is vitally important, and by reasonable standards it has, so far, been a success. But why should the government leap so quickly into the AIDS arena when it is so callous to the needs of more than 2,500 who will die this and every year, needlessly, from breast and cervical cancer because they were not screened in time?

Could the answer be that health is a political issue? Could it be that the government primarily spends money to defend its own survival, and not to defend survival of the population? AIDS is a new pandemic which has caught all countries by surprise. Early efforts to combat it can only improve the government's reputation. By contrast, breast and cervical cancer are established killers. Any focus on screening programmes exposes only the gap between the UK and enlightened countries like Sweden, Iceland and Finland. It reveals that the government has effectively condemned thousands of women because it has been too miserly to protect them from preventable death.

Region and Class

Great regional disparities in health exist,[62] as they have done since the 1950s. In Wales, for instance, death from heart disease and strokes in men of all social classes is much higher than in the rest of the UK,[63] and has been for at least 20 years.[64] Accordingly, an Oxfordshire man born in the early 1970s can expect to live until his 71st birthday. But if he had been born in Wales, less than 70 miles away, he could expect to die three years earlier at 68.[65] If social class is added into the equation, the working class Welshman will be lucky to reach his 66th birthday, while the toff in Oxford can expect to live until he is 73.

These gross inequalities expose the failure of the government to narrow the health gap between north and south, rich and poor. Indeed, when evidence emerged that the gap was actually widening, the government made every effort to suppress it. The Black Report was submitted to the Secretary of State in April 1980. But instead of publishing it under the stamp of the DHSS or the HMSO, the government chose to bury its findings. Only 260 duplicated copies of the typescript were made available and they were released when they would receive the least media attention – in the week of the August bank holiday. Major organizations within the NHS, including health authorities, did not even receive copies.[66]

The present government can hardly be blamed for the state of the national health as captured by the Black report at the beginning of 1980 when it had only been in power for a few months. But seven years later, when it was entirely account-able, it chose again to suppress publication of the follow-up report, *The Health Divide*, in 1987. The new report[67] also showed the strong relationship between illness and poverty in Britain. Moreover, it showed that the health gap between the poor and wealthy had continued to widen since the 1980 Black Report.[68] And it revealed that many of the key recommen-dations of the earlier report, which might have helped reverse the trend, had been studiously ignored.

On the day that *The Health Divide* was due to be published, the chairman of the Health Education Council denied any knowledge of its existence. This later proved to be untrue. But he cancelled the press launch and instructed the director of the Council, Dr David Player, not to speak to the media, and attempted to withdraw all copies of the report. This unseemly attempt at censorship failed, but only because it was so badly bungled. An impromptu press conference was held, in hastily borrowed accommodation in Soho, London, and the report was finally released without deletions.

'Chemical Comforters' – Legal, Lethal, Drug Abuse

The government will not spend money to prevent disease. It will not effectively regulate the drug industry to control its profits or to clamp down on its worthless products and misleading claims. But perhaps the clearest evidence of all that the government is a double agent – promoting its own interests at the expense of the national health – is its failure to control the alcohol and tobacco industries.

These two poisons cause immense misery by way of disease and death each year. Add up the financial cost: diseases related to smoking cost the NHS £200 million each year and alcohol related diseases cost a further £100 million. Days of lost work, caused by drinking, cost industry another £640 million a year.

Having counted cash, let's count bodies. Alcohol directly kills 8,000 each year in the UK and contributes to the death of another 1200 through loss of coordination and control – the number of road deaths and murders reckoned to be drink related.[69]

Alcohol is but a plaything compared to tobacco. Smoking is directly responsible for the death of 100,000 each year in the UK. And it is now recognized that even non-smokers face increased risk of disease and death from living in a smoke-polluted atmosphere. The risk of a non-smoker dying of lung cancer is increased by a factor of 1.3 if he or she is living with one person smoking twenty or more cigarettes a day, and by 2.3 if living with two.

Current trends show that smoking is declining for most segments of society, although not, unfortunately, for young women between the ages of 16 and 19. But the trend for alcohol is very different. It shows that since the early 1980s alcohol consumption in the UKKhas increased by about 6% per year, although much of the increase may, again, be attributed to more drinking by the young and especially girls.

Governments constantly argue that they are doing all they can to restrict the use of these chemical comforters. This is not true. Successive governments have skirted around the real issues because they do not want to face unpopularity at the polls, they value the jobs which the cigarette and alcohol industries provide and they enjoy enormously the revenues which the two industries bring in from duty on their products. So, the government pays only lip service to controlling alcohol and tobacco. The health warning on every packet is still only a voluntary arrangement between government and the industry. Written advertising by the tobacco industry is controlled, again in a voluntary fashion, by the Advertising Standards Authority. Exclusion of cigarette advertising from television is implemented by the Independent Broadcasting Association.

Straddling all these arrangements is the Committee for Monitoring Agreements on Tobacco Adverting and Sponsorship which was set up in December 1986 and has an independent chair and members drawn from the departments of health (England, Scotland and Northern Ireland) and from representatives of the Tobacco Advisory Council and Imported Tobacco Products Advisory Council. These informal arrangements provide a semblance of control. The real truth is that government only provides £2.7 million each year toward anti-drink education and not much more, £3.5 million, on information designed to stop people from smoking. Of course, these sums are dwarfed by the sums which the tobacco and alcohol industries spend on advertising and promotion. The alcohol industry spends £200 million a year in Britain on promotion. And the tobacco industry, even though it is largely barred from television advertising, still manages to spend £100 million a year. A government education programme costing about one fiftieth of this amount is clearly inadequate. Indeed there is evidence, as we have already seen, that the government will actively suppress those, including its own agents, who speak out for the national health.

Under Dr David Player's direction, the Health Education Council was also a fierce critic of the alcohol and tobacco industries. In March 1987 he was dismissed and the Council's terms of reference were altered by the government, so that it is effectively neutered in future debates. The HEC showed itself to be fearless and independent, and it paid the price.

No government, it seems, has been prepared to risk losing votes by curbing the use of alcohol and tobacco. Nor is any government prepared to lose its duty income. In 1985–86 the Exchequer received £4.05 billion from cigarette sales and £6.26 billion from the sale of alcohol.[70] The jobs which the two industries provide, especially in politically sensitive areas, must also be considered. The government gives grants to the Northern Ireland tobacco industry of £3.5 million each year – exactly the same sum that it spends on its entire anti-smoking campaign.[71] The government even gave at least

£1 million to an American Tobacco company to set up an ill-fated factory for making, and marketing, a nicotine chewing gum even though specialists warned that the product would cause cancer. The factory was closed last year.

If the government is then a double agent, concerned merely to defend its revenue and to sponsor the drug, alcohol and tobacco industries, who remains to defend the national health?

The answer is that enlightened doctors and informed people must fight together. It will not be an easy battle. The government's commitment to secrecy and to keeping power over health is total. In the next chapter we look at ways in which the public at large can become successfully involved in the health debate. Ultimately it will be patients, as voters, who will change the system.

CHAPTER 4
Patient Heal Thyself

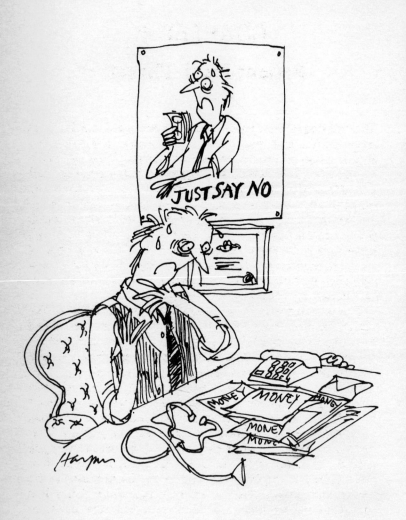

CHAPTER 4

Patient Heal Thyself

The message from opinion polls is clear – the public cares about health, and cares more about it than anything else. Health is uppermost on the public agenda. It is the public who are the consumers, it is the public who get ill, who fund the NHS, and who actually take the medicines. Yet here is the paradox. The public, as patients, are the least well informed in the health debate. They are seldom consulted about health policy. And at the sharp end, when they enter the doctor's surgery they are weak, indeed impotent. They have little or no say in their treatment. And should they dare to show any intelligent interest in their own bodies, most doctors see them as a threat and adversary, rather than as an ally.

The paradox is not only illogical, it is also malign. The patient, ill and frightened, stands alone against the unified front of providers – the politicians, the drug industry and the doctors, who often have a greater interest in protecting each other than they do in advancing the national health.

How can the public confront this combined power? How can patients assert their rights over their own therapy, over the prescription pad, over their own fate? After all, most medical treatment consists of doctors prescribing drugs. How can we, as patients, wrest the power of the prescribing pen from the prejudice of the medical establishment who use it to protect their own privilege? This is the battlefront, in the surgery and in the ballot box. Patients must assert themselves and stand up to their own physicians and they must, as voters, demand that the drug industry serves them before its shareholders.

The public remains, however, excluded from its rightful position in the centre of the health debate. Patients will gain this ground when they are better informed and they begin to assert themselves. Equity will be achieved when they can argue and lobby from positions of strength, to persuade government that secrecy is against the public interest, that greater consultation and participation with patients will strengthen the decision-making process and make the NHS more effective.

Pressure groups, in all shapes and sizes, have an important part to play. It is easy to dismiss local support groups, consisting of a few patients and friends who fight against a grievance, but they have an uncanny habit of growing into national campaigns – such as the Terence Higgins Trust for AIDS victims, Mind and Mencap for patients with mental disability, and Action For Smoking and Health (ASH). These consumer movements have forced the health providers to rethink their public positions. The British Medical Association has recently published critical articles on the problems of growing old, the unjustifiable hazards of boxing, drugs in the 3rd World and the long-term effects of nuclear war. Even the drugs industry, in the slippery guise of its think tank – the Office of Health Economics (OHE) – has published articles on AIDS, multiple sclerosis and women's health. Each of these is helpful and suggests a real realignment of thinking. But we should not be seduced too easily. When the author of the OHE pamphlet on women's health was asked why he failed to mention that women take a disproportionate amount of the drugs prescribed, he replied, without conviction, that this was an unintentional oversight.

Public debates which influence new legislation must always be welcome, particularly in controlling the worst promotional abuses of the drug industry. But real changes in the therapeutic dialogue will occur only when the atmosphere between doctor and patient fundamentally alters in the consulting room. An atmosphere where doctor and patient enjoy mutual respect, where they recognize each others needs, rights and limitations, and where they work together toward a common goal. If this is ever to come about, patients have obligations as well as rights. They have a responsibility to understand their disease. They have an obligation to understand and share in their treatment. They must also play a part in the advancement of medicine. This means they should volunteer to participate in drug trials. And they must, as citizens, campaign to control the drug industry so that its enormous benefits are harnessed to serve patients before profits and shareholders.

Heal Thyself: Understanding Disease

People view their health in terms of how, through their senses, they feel. We use the term 'perfect health' – indeed it is top in the classification used by the World Health Organization. In reality, however, it is a misnomer, a myth. There is no such thing as perfect health – not least because, as living creatures getting older, we are all dying slowly.

Most of us spend most of our time claiming to be in good health even when we are feeling vaguely unwell and taking remedies. Surveys here shown that headaches, sore throats, stomach aches and lassitude are all so common that even people who describe themselves as well will have at least one such symptom and take at least one medicine to deal with it every week.[1,2]. At what point do they join the 12% of us whose ill health restricts our activity[3] or forces us to visit a GP, as each of us does, about four times a year?[4]

It is when we fall into poor health that the fear and the conflict begin. Unable to cope or function properly, we are driven to the doctor in search of a diagnosis and cure. We feel ill, and we want the doctor to confirm our suspicions in a way that doesn't frighten us to death. Both sides are under pressure. We as patients want answers. Doctors are expected to find instant, reassuring solutions.

As patients we feel 'symptoms'. The doctor, however, cannot personally experience these. He or she can only observe 'signs'. In order to understand more, for example, about a patient complaining of a sore knee, the doctor asks a series of questions. How long has it hurt; did it follow an accident; does the joint feel warm; does it swell; is there relief if the joint in put in a particular position; does it keep you awake at night; do you feel ill in any other way?

The answers build a picture of the illness, telling the doctor what should be examined, what special tests may be needed to corroborate the patient's story. They may also throw up clues that even the patient has not noticed. Enlargement of the lymph glands in the groin is an obvious indication of likely infection. Diagnosis is not always so straightforward. That painful knee may actually be the result of damage to the patient's heart valves. And the clue may actually be discovered in telltale signs in the finger nails! Certain kinds of heart valve infection (subacute bacterial endocarditis) can spread infection throughout the body. The infection can land in the knee joint. For reasons that we still don't understand, people with this infection will also have swollen ends to their finger tips and the curves to their finger nails become exaggerated in a characteristic manner.

If a patient's history, subsequent examination and corroborating tests (x-rays, blood analysis, biopsy, body scans etc) are all positive and pointing in the same direction, then the diagnosis is fairly easily made. For example, if the patient complains of passing excessive amounts of urine (history), if the blood vessels at the back of the patient's eye show characteristic swelling (examination) and blood tests show that the level of blood sugar is raised, then it is certain that the patient is suffering from sugar diabetes.

Things are not always this straightforward. What if the doctor can find nothing from examination or laboratory tests to confirm the symptoms felt by a patient? For some conditions, like depression or schizophrenia, there are no physical tests to confirm the problem. Diagnostic tests may also be used inappropriately. A chest x-ray obviously won't help diagnose diabetes, nor will a blood test reveal the existence of lung cancer.

Communication, built on trust between patient and doctor, becomes extremely important when the cluster of symptoms remains baffling. The trouble is that even well-meaning and open patients can be poor witnesses to their own complaints. Patients tend to forget or dismiss symptoms if they are no real threat. Who can remember, for example, how many headaches they had last month or when they suffered their last bout of diarrhoea unless these symptoms caused disabling pain and/or acute embarrassment? A sore throat to an opera singer or an aching ankle to a footballer would almost certainly cause anxiety. If, however, the symptoms were swapped neither would rush to the surgery for a remedy or even, perhaps, remember the incident. A woman with abdominal pain will interpret her condition quite differently if she is pregnant, or merely expecting her monthly menstrual period.

In addition, the brain can compound or reduce symptoms of illness. Most enlightened doctors now accept that there is no clear distinction between physical illness and psychologically induced disease. The sensation of shortness of breath may be quite out of proportion to the actual physical disturbance that can be seen in the lungs. Anxiety will visibly increase an existing rash. We now know that acute mental stress can actually weaken the body's immune system. Equally, weeks of pain, tenderness, depression and fatigue arising from a suspected tumour can disappear within seconds when a patient learns that the tests for cancer turned out, after all, to be negative.

The psyche may do even more than merely react to (and enhance or diminish) a physical insult. It can lead and orchestrate disease. It can be the primary seat of the condition. In a patient with schizophrenia or depression, there is no physical pointer, no certain chemical imbalance, to diagnose the condition.

There is something very attractive about the idea that treatment, and so the drugs that are prescribed, should be symptom-led. Symptoms are the key component which patients bring to the relation with doctors. They are at the core of communication and doctors who overlook or disregard patients' symptoms, as many clearly do,[5] should be condemned for their negligence.

There is need, though, for considerable caution. Doctors have been trained, quite correctly, to look beyond or behind evident symptoms. They can often detect disease or abnormality of which patients are still unaware – for example high blood pressure – which needs urgent treatment. Second, the whole field of preventive medicine (immunization, cervical screening, and so on) is designed to keep people healthy and symptom-free. Third, many patients – the unborn, the severely mentally handicapped and the unconscious – cannot communicate the symptoms they feel. Here the doctor is obliged to be in command of treatment.

The whole 'whose-body-is-it-anyway?' dilemma is easily illustrated. Consider a patient admitted by ambulance to casualty suffering from a suspected and intentional drugs overdose. While the patient remains conscious the doctor is expected to honour the convention that the swallowed poisons should not be removed without the patient's permission. And yet, as soon as the patient lapses into unconsciousness, unimpeded resuscitation can begin. The stomach can be emptied of the offending drug and the patient allowed – or in some cases obliged against his or her will – to recover.

Even when a patient is intelligent, alert and cooperative, symptoms still remain an imperfect guide to treatment. They are a subjective, highly personal view of illness. It is impossible for a patient to judge the true medical significance of the symptoms they think they feel. They are influenced by their own psychological states and imperfect memories.

One of my patients recently told me of a most frightening episode in which he suddenly became dizzy and collapsed, fearing that he was dying. Certain aspects of the illness puzzled me. It was important to find out whether he had ever experienced such symptoms before. The patient was adamant, absolutely convinced that this was his first and only attack. And yet, to my surprise I saw in his notes an account of an almost identical episode with the same symptoms only three years earlier. Why did he conceal this, or did he genuinely forget? And if he forgot, was it the fear of staring death in the face that caused him completely to black out the memory? Alternatively, was it all make-believe? Was he simply enjoying the attention of being whisked to hospital and made a fuss of by a sympathetic doctor? The only sure thing is that I remain confused about the quality of his evidence. But two incidents, even if apocryphal, must be investigated. Clues from his heart trace suggested that his turns were real, that they originated in his heart and are amenable to treatment.

Patients also modify their behaviour, quite unconsciously and slowly over time, to accommodate their disease. Elderly patients with chronic lung disease purse their lips in almost identical fashion. The reason they do this is that they have learned, unconsciously, to balance the pressures inside and outside their chests in an effort to improve their breathing and reduce their disability. As a simple method of treatment, it works reasonably well. The same instinct for self-treatment and survival occurs in young children born with a condition known as Fallot's tetralogy, a complex deformity of the heart including holes in the heart's chambers and abnormalities in its valves. The result is that blood fails to flow freely to the lungs to be reoxygenated. The children unconsciously learn to squat in a characteristic posture which helps to force the blood up through the lungs.

Inevitably, too, serious illness will impair judgement even in the most level-headed and resilient patient. One of the most vulnerable times for an asthmatic is just when he or she is beginning to recover after a serious attack. They fail to recognize the severity of their disability and are prone to over exert themselves while neglecting vital medication. I have seen such ill-judged overconfidence kill patients who were released from hospital too soon.

Doctors can try to measure a patient's symptoms against some independent measure of normality. If a little girl of four develops severe abdominal pain and vaginal bleeding she is almost certainly ill. If she were nine, these symptoms would be seen as an early but normal menstrual period requiring only the sympathetic reassurance of parents and teachers. Yet the same symptoms in a nine-year-old of the 1940s would have caused anxiety and medical attention since the onset of menstruation in that generation did not usually begin before the age of 14. Now, if a healthy and well-nourished girl did not have her first period by the age of 16 this would give cause for concern – unless, of course, she was a gymnast or other highly trained athlete whose intense exercise schedule delayed her normal onset of periods.

The pattern of illness also affects the assertiveness of individual patients. When only mildly ill, most patients put the highest store on their own symptoms and are most assertive in determining what treatment they expect to get. But as they become more ill, they become less assertive and more compliant – wanting, as their fear grows, to hand more and more of the responsibility for their healing to their doctor. On most occasions this shifting of responsibility occurs by tacit agreement and is of mutual advantage. But too many doctors still find initially assertive patients a nuisance and an annoying threat to their authority. This clash is never more obvious than when an old-fashioned consultant obstetrician meets an intelligent, assertive and entirely healthy young woman who happens to be pregnant. She is robust in her belief that as the mother of the unborn child inside her womb she has an active role to play – indeed the primary role – in deciding the prenatal care that she and the child will receive. Here the sparks begin to fly. A consult of the old school is the oracle of all medical wisdom: any unsolicited utterances, questions or opinions from mothers-to-be are a waste of his valuable time.

The women's movement, having taken its lead from the United States, has begun to fight for the rights of female patients, and especially pregnant women. It and other patient pressure groups have begun to challenge the whole ritual of medical mystification that leaves patients weak and uninformed. To many doctors this sort of patients rights campaign is a threat. Assertive patients are not welcome in their consulting rooms. To a growing minority of doctors – and here I include myself – such assertiveness is refreshing and even challenging and we hope it will grow. More than 10% of my outpatients now come to the clinic accompanied by well companions who aid them in getting a fair hearing. These companions are my allies too. They can offer clues about the patient's illness and are likely to know whether the patient will stay on the course of treatment I recommend. Decisions on treatment must take this kind of 'pastoral' information into account.[6] This brigade of accompanying friends can be awkward, ill-informed and meddlesome. But let us hope that they are here to stay – almost as public inspectors – for they will undoubtedly change methods of medical practice.

Doctors and Diagnosis

Confidence in diagnosis would be so much greater if doctors were differently trained and selected. As we have seen, it is no accident that most doctors are white, male and middle-class. Moreover, the position is unlikely to change quickly since racial discrimination during admission to medical schools was still standard in 1986[7] and although discrimination against women seems less at this stage, it starts for them soon after qualifying.

The values generally held by white middle-class males are not always shared by the poor, the underprivileged, women and members of the ethnic minorities. Is it any real surprise that these groups are so often fobbed off with excessive and inappropriate prescriptions of valium and other mood-changing drugs? It is so much easier to prescribe a hypnotic drug to a working-class black woman than to risk trying to understand and solve her underlying problems. It is no coincidence either that opinion surveys repeatedly describe doctors as aloof, overbearing, distant, disinterested, dismissive, frightening and engendering feelings of guilt in the patient. Indeed, doctors seem a very difficult group to get on with.[8]

Treatment in Tandem

If patients want to be active partners in the therapeutic dialogue, then they must also be prepared to share some of the responsibilities of treatment. They must take an active interest in which drugs they are prescribed, and even more, they must be prepared to participate in the research that provides the very data that they, themselves, seek. So far, only a rare few have campaigned for greater involvement of patients in their own care, and I suspect that the majority of people may always seek to decline any responsibility for their own medical welfare. Many patients do not even know the name and nature of the disease from which they are suffering, and nor do they wish to remember any important details of their treatment beyond what colour their tablets are.

I suspect that much of this apparent lack of interest is a disguise. It is part of the deeply rooted process of denial which so shapes our attitude toward disease and death. Whatever the motive, the behaviour gives many arrogant doctors an excuse to label many of their patients as ignorant and to justify their failure to communicate.

Doctors have always been part of the Health Conspiracy. Since serious treatment began they have chosen to make patients feel passive and dependent. They have kept their methods secret, resisted telling patients the results of their diagnoses, and have failed to give the names of the medicines they prescribe. Not only is their handwriting frequently illegible but they still have the right to prescribe in Latin, to obfuscate their message even further, if they choose.

Recent attempts to arm the patient with information have not been very successful. Most of the more sensitive and useful information which doctors hold on their patients cannot be obtained under the Data Protection Act. Although the Act gives access to records held on computer, doctors can refuse to disclose information on the grounds that it would be harmful to patients. Also, the Act does not require doctors (or anyone else) to disclose opinions they might hold. So if your GP thinks your lifestyle makes you a likely target for AIDS, you have no right to know about it. Furthermore, most GP's records are not yet on computer file, and are therefore specifically excluded from the Act.

The one real ray of hope has been the passage of the Access to Medical Reports Act – a private member's bill that was pushed through parliament by the Liberal MP Archie Kirkwood in July 1988 . It requires doctors to disclose to patients a copy of the medical report which they send to insurance companies and employers. There are exclusions. The government insisted on an amendment to protect national security – which means that soldiers, Ministry of Defence workers and even employees of Sellafield may be unable to find out their exposure to radioactivity. But ordinary people will at least be able to discover whether their doctor thinks they are a bad insurance or work risk and the reasons why.

The Obligation to Inform

On moral grounds alone, doctors have an obligation to inform their patients about the kind of treatment they are administering. Medicines cause side effects in 10% of the people who take them. Some are severe, others less so; all are worrying to the recipient.

The anti-tuberculosis drug ethambutol can, for example, cause blindness. It is reversible and normal sight can be fully restored if the drug is stopped quickly enough. But I know of at least one patient in the UK who went permanently blind from the drug in 1987 because he had not been warned about the adverse reaction, and told what to do, by the hospital doctor. The GP could have helped if he'd been told that the ethambutol was being prescribed, but no such information arrived.

In Britain patients almost never resort to the courts to pursue a claim for medical negligence. Litigation with the frequency and level of reward seen in the United States may not, on the other hand, be a goal to be aimed at either. As the Opren case showed (see Chapter 2), proving negligence against a drug company can be very difficult and the eventual level of compensation derisory. Claims against doctors for medical negligence have been more successful and the level of award, in many cases, substantially higher.

Doctors actually have some legal duty to inform patients about the risks of therapy, although their obligations are shaped (or kept relatively indistinct) by case law rather than by precise statute.[9] Doctors have a basic obligation to ensure that patients have all the information they need to enable them to decide whether or not to take a partticular medicine. However, case law suggests that if a patient requests no information then a doctor can get away with offering minimal advice. If an assertive patient demands to know the precise risks of treatment, then the doctor is obliged to explain in detail to avoid any suggestion of negligence.[10]

Most doctors seem still to prefer their patients to be quiet, passive and compliant – people who will do what they are told, take their medicines without question and reliably follow instructions. This level of domination may massage the ego of arrogant physicians, but it is positively dangerous to the national health. It is wretched to discover patients who have got progressively iller – not from a disease, but from the side effects of medication – and yet who were too timid or intimidated to question their treatment and stop swallowing the tablets.

Positive Practice: Patients Take the Lead

Ideally, every patient should play an active, even vociferous role in treatment. This begins with understanding their own symptoms, and it continues with their determination to see the doctor as just the provider of another modern service. 'My body isn't working as it should, and they tell me you are qualified to fix it. How do you propose to go about it?'

Many patients will, because they are passive and fearful, abrogate this responsibility. The process of denial – the desire to escape responsibility when the prospect of pain and death looms – is too great. I want to see a programme of action for those patients who will fight, who will play an active role and thereby contribute effectively to their own treatment. They will tell their doctor about the previous drug reactions they have had, or even the reactions that close relatives have suffered, because some reactions are inherited. When taking a drug they will volunteer to monitor its performance and report any unsuspected reactions, not just for themselves but for others, because unrecognized, the drug's side effects could be harming large numbers of people.

Patients who take an active part in their own therapy can also be less expensive. Studies show that passive patients, who little understand their treatment, never bother to get their prescriptions from the chemist, and those who do rarely finish the prescribed course. Untold money and energy are lost simply because patients lack confidence in their own therapy.

More active patients would also demand better labelling of the medicines they were prescribed. The Pharmaceutical Society deserves credit for bringing standards up to the reasonable levels we have achieved. Each prescription label must bear the name of the patient, the name and address of the supplier, the date of dispensing, basic warnings like 'keep out of the reach of children' and 'for external use only', directions for use and precautions requested by the prescriber. Current legislation also requires that labels should be mechanically printed, to avoid the confusion of hand writing. Pharmacists are also encouraged to add at least one of 28 stock, cautionary phrases which they have all committed to memory like 'Do not stop this medicine except on your doctor's advice'.

The system assumes, though, that all prescribed drugs are essentially benevolent. This is both false and naïve. Drug companies produce a vast array of tranquillizers, not because they wish particularly to benefit public health, but because they wish to maximize profits for their shareholders. Equally, doctors prescribe them, not necessarily because they are seeking the optimum solution to patients' problems, but because the prescription is the easiest way to get an anxious patient out of the surgery. Nowhere in Britain will you see on a bottle of tranquillizers the obvious health warning: 'Caution: this medicine can cause dependence'.

Equally, there are no laws to require patient pack inserts – longer pamphlets of information, written in a readable style, to inform patients about the drugs they are taking.[11] The Association of the British Pharmaceutical Industry recently agreed, in yet another voluntary code of practice, to make them universally available. This is another case of allowing the poacher to set the rules on behalf of the gamekeeper. The ABPI will have control over the contents and style of all patient pack inserts. We have already seen how poorly the ABPI performs in policing its own members when they falsely promote drugs to doctors. Should we expect any higher standards from drug companies when they will have the opportunity to put their message to patients directly? Can we expect them to concur in the sensible suggestion that they put warning black triangles on the patient pack inserts of all new drugs? This would alert patients to be especially aware of adverse reactions. Recent attempts to use this simple warning system have been met with silence.[12, 13]

Alternative Information

Where else should patients turn for informed, yet dispassionate information about medicines, if both their own doctors and the industry lack candour and concern? Many pharmacists, long trained in the behaviour of drugs, can be a reliable source of help, even if they cannot replace the advice and knowledge of doctors. Patient lobbies and pressure groups, albeit occasionally misinformed or ill-informed, also play a most useful role. And it is important that the lay media, which so often come under attack, are praised for the very useful job they do. Some of the most effective advice recently on AIDS and drug abuse has come not from doctors, the government or the drug industry, but from television, the radio and the serious newspapers.

Early attempts by the media to probe serious medical matters prompted, perhaps not surprisingly, a stern reaction from the medical and governmental establishment. When the BBC began its mould-breaking series, *Your Life in Their Hands* in 1958, the *British Medical Journal* heaped scorn on the programme,[14] and participants to the programme were warned, *sotto voce*, that their medical careers had been jeopardised by their public display.[15] Even now the medical establishment regards the lay media with caution and scepticism. Of course, the lay media have made mistakes. I think they have been excessively harsh in their criticism of the whooping cough vaccine. The vaccine may in rare cases, cause horrific brain damage, but the disease itself can leave horrendous handicap or cause death. No one was growing very rich out of the whooping cough vaccine, and for a product so much in the medical balance, it was subjected to insensitive attack. BBC's *Panorama* programme may well have done long term public good by exposing some of the less savory aspects of the organ transplant industry, but in the way it was handled the net effect was virtually to cut off the supply of donated organs for a time.

Medical coverage in the tabloid press is often flippant, meddling and not worthy of further comment. The serious lay media have persisted in producing outstanding investigative programmes on medical issues. On television, *Panorama*, *World in Action*, *Horizon*, and the Channel 4 series *Kill or Cure* have all pushed back the frontiers of understanding. So have the BBC Radio 4 programmes, *Medicine Now* and *File-on-Four*. Specialist correspondents with a genuine regard for the ethical issues at stake have emerged. They include Geoff Watts of BBC radio, Andy Veitch of ITN, and James Erlichman, Annabel Ferriman, Oliver Gillie and Nick Timmins of the serious press.

Drug Trials: Your Mouth Where Their Money Is

If patients are serious in their desire to take an active role in therapy, then they must volunteer to advance treatment by taking part in drug trials. Naturally, all of us are frightened to be involved in experimental trials. No one wants to be a guinea pig, especially when reassurances from doctors cannot be trusted. As we have seen in chapter 2, volunteers can be injured and, in extreme cases, even die from adverse drug reactions. But these events are, it must be stressed, very rare. It is almost certainly safer to take part in a drug trial than to drive from Lands End to John O'Groats.

There are risks, however, and they are bigger than they need be. Drug companies have no obvious obligation to maintain the most rigorous safety standards. Volunteers have no automatic right to compensation if things go wrong, and the chances that the mistakes of the trial will be exposed by publicity are remote. The local ethical committees ought to have the muscle to guarantee safe protocols. Unfortunately, they lack the statutory power to exert their authority.

Civic duty aside, there is no point in volunteering for a trial, if the drug under test is virtually worthless, or the study is merely a disguised sales exercise to increase the drug's market share. The only safeguards a volunteer has are these: he or she should ask the doctor in charge, 'Does this study have ethical committee approval and would you yourself risk your health to take part in it?'

Compensation

People injured in drug trials should not have to face the laborious task of fighting huge pharmaceutical companies through the courts in search of compensation. They have risked themselves not only for the national health, but in the end, for the company's profits. Compensation, in the case of injury, should be immediate, uncomplicated and generous, yet, this hardly ever occurs. Volunteers, be they healthy or patients, have no more rights in law than ordinary patients, like the victims of thalidomide or Opren, who are innocently injured by the side effects of drugs.

For everyone who receives medicines there should be no-fault compensation if the drug has caused serious injury. Many schemes have been suggested. The easiest seems a levy on drug company profits (based on sales) which would go into a central kitty. The compensation scheme already operated in Sweden seems particularly attractive. It clearly recognizes risks and levels of injury and is being energetically supported as a model for the UK by the British Medical Association.

Much needs to be campaigned for before we can enjoy a just drugs policy in Britain. What follows is a prescription for improving the public's health.

CHAPTER 5
The Prescription

"*I'll need your cooperation for this course of treatment Miss Miller –
could you read your way towards me?*"

CHAPTER 5

The Prescription

The national health will not improve until patients demand a greater role in the provision of their own treatment. This will not be easy. Doctors, as we have seen, jealously guard their privileges. The drug industry jealousy guards its profits, and the government, for reasons of its own, behaves as a double agent, on the one hand protecting the drugs industry and on the other being responsible for regulating the use of medicines by the public.

The health providers, doctors, the drug industry and government, use the shroud of secrecy to keep the public powerless and in the dark. The prescription for change is not a matter of increasing health expenditure or choosing a particular party to form a government. There will need to be a new alliance between patients and providers. Patients have faced a Health Conspiracy in which their interests and those of the public at large, have been subservient to the providers. For this mould to be broken and a new one formed, the first priority must be for each group to put its own house in order; to develop practices that champion the health of all members of the community. This done a merger between alll four groups should be possible.

Changes are essential if we hope to provide a health service equal to that of other countries of similar wealth.

The Pharmaceutical Industry

• The pharmaceutical industry must recognize that its marketing and promotional practices are essentially untenable and will be exposed when doctors and patients regain control over treatment.

• Profits are legitimate when they are earned from valuable

and innovative drugs which reduce illness and patient suffering. Profits must be increasingly condemned when they are earned from 'me-too' medicines and from over-promotion of outdated and unneeded products. Profits will also be increasingly ridiculed when they are won at the expense of cheaper, generic alternatives.

• Scientists working in the industry must remember that their first duty is to science; doctors that their first duty is to patients. They must resist marketing pressures designed to force their research into areas unlikely to improve health or unlikely to contribute to real understanding. They must feel responsible if the medicines they develop are over-promoted or when side effects are ignored, minimized or obscured.

• The marketing and promotional side of the industry must curb their ways so that advertisements are legible, honest, and factually correct.

The Government

• The government must separate its support for the drug industry from that of controlling its profits and abuses. Commercial sponsorship of the industry must be handed over to the Department of Trade and Industry.

• Regulation of the industry must be strengthened under the newly proposed Medicines Directorate at the Department of Health. Efforts by the drug industry to direct the new watchdog body should be fiercely resisted.

• The Medicines Act requires fundamental revision. This must include:

    a) An end to the secrecy which prevents doctors, patients and the responsible media from uncovering unhealthy links between government and industry; which allows incompetence within the division to remain hidden; and which permits dangerous or useless drugs to be marketed.

    b) New rules on the licensing of drugs which would require pharmaceutical companies to give verifiable evidence of genuine clinical efficacy for all new discoveries. But even this is not enough. The law

152

must prevent the marketing of new drugs unless they can be shown to provide therapeutic benefit superior to that of existing products. Drugs should only be licensed if there is proven clinical need for them. This will inevitably lead to the extension of the limited list across all therapeutic categories and the legal requirements for pharmacists to substitute cheaper, generic drugs wherever and whenever available.

c) Patients must be guaranteed the right to receive full and readable information with every prescription.

d) All expert advisers to the government must be required to publicly declare their financial and professional connections with the pharmaceutical industry.

e) Volunteers in drug trials should enjoy complete legal protection and compensation in the event of injury.

f) Clinical trials must not be undertaken without prior approval from a properly constituted ethical committee. The licensing authority should not accept manufacturer's data without evidence of such approval.

● The new Medicines Directorate must have the powers, the resources and the will to implement the Act. It must increase the size, competence and activities of its staff so as to provide a more thorough control of licensing and relicensing of medicines, and of drug company advertising and promotion. The directorate should be prepared to lead, responding to public concern as much as to pressures from doctors and the industry.
● Government should increase its support for medical research. Neglected areas such as prevention, complementary medicine and non-drug therapy need much fuller resourcing.
● Government should establish a 'no-fault' compensation scheme to cover all patients who suffer medical injury.
● Profits earned by the drug industry under the Pharmaceut-

ical Price Regulation Scheme should be exposed in detail to public scrutiny.

• Government should establish a list of patients' rights which all those involved in health provision should respect.

• The government should ensure that health policies are applied equally and fully throughout the NHS with no geographical area, ethnic group, gender or class being disadvantaged.

Doctors

There must be a public inquiry to examine the selection of students to medical schools. Racism, sexism and classism, where it exists, must be eradicated. Selection criteria should be reassessed and the current practice of giving priority to academic achievement reconsidered – alternative qualities might be more relevant.

• The General Medical Council, the body responsible for training doctors, must become more open to public scrutiny and more sensitive to public demand. It should ensure that medical education trains doctors to serve the interests of patients – it should not exist to protect the interests of the medical establishment.

• Doctors, as painful as it may be to their egos, must recognize that they exist to prevent illness and to treat patients when they are ill. Medical training must reflect this humility and humanity. Treatment must be an equal partnership.

• Doctors must become much more vigilant in their dealings with the pharmaceutical industry. They must see that there can often be an essential conflict between their job of serving patients and the drug industry's job of maximizing profits for shareholders. There are many alternative therapies, some radical and some conventional, which do not require the prescription pad. Above all, doctors themselves must campaign for more preventive medicine within the health service.

Patients

- Patients must recognize that they have the power for change.
- They must take greater responsibility for their own treatment by asserting their rights in the surgery. This includes greater vigilance in taking medicines and reporting adverse reactions when they occur.
- They must take a greater and more active role in research as volunteers in clinical experiments.
- As citizens they must, in pressure groups and at the ballot box, demand that government serves them above the doctors, the drug industry or its own self-interest. This must include their right, as consumers of treatment, to sit on ethical committees, regional health authorities and all major medical review bodies.

These changes will not come easily or without pain. But everything in the agenda can be achieved within the existing framework of the National Health Service. If the integrity of the NHS is destroyed, then nothing can be achieved. Britain has the makings of the finest medical service in the world at the lowest possible price. If we could all work together to the common goal of patient welfare then the ideal of health for all by the year 2000 is in our grasp.

References

Chapter 1: Practice Imperfect

1. Reynolds, M., 'No news is bad news; patients' views about communication in hospital', *British Medical Journal*, 1978; 1: 1673–1676.

2. Fitton, F. and Acheson, H. W., *The doctor/patient relationship: a study in general practice*, HMSO, London, 1979.

3. *Inequalities in Health:* Report of the Working Group on Inequalities in Health chaired by Sir Douglas Black. DHSS, 1980.

4. *Heart Beat Wales, 1987; 7: Pulse of Wales*. Published by Heart Beat Wales, 1987.

5. *The Health Divide*, Health Education Council, London, March, 1987.

6. Le Grand J., 'Inequalities in Health and Health care: a research agenda', *Class and Health*, edited by Richard G. Wilkinson. Tavistock Publications, London, 1986.

7. Pendleton, D. A. and Bochner, S., 'The Communication of medical information in general Practice consultations as a function of patient's social class,' *Social Science and Medicine*, 1980; 14: 669–673. See also: Bain, D. J. G., 'Doctor patient communication in general practice consultations', *Medical Education*, 1976; 10; 125–131.

8. Bain, D. J. G. 'Patient Knowledge and the content of the consultation in general practice', *Medical Education*, 1977; 11: 347–350.

9. Blaxter, M., 'Equity and Consultation rates in General Practice', *British Medical Journal*, 1984; 288: 1963–1967.

10. McManus, I. C., 'The Social Class of Medical Students', *Medical Education*, 1982; 16:72–75.

11. 'Medical and dental staffing prospects in the NHS in England and Wales,' *Health Trends*, 1987; 19:1–8.

12. Leeson, J. and Gray. J., *Women and Medicine*, Tavistock Publications, London, 1978.

156

13. *On the State of the Public Health for the Year*, HMSO, London, 1983.

14. Collier, J. G. and Burke, A., 'Racial and sexual discrimination in the selection of students for London medical Schools,' *Medical Education*, 1986; 20:86–90.

15. *Medical School Admissions: Report of a Formal Investigation into St George's Hospital Medical School*, Published by The Commission For Racial Equality, London, 1988.

16. Hansard, *Written Answers*, 29 Feb, Column 405, 1988.

17. Allen, I., *Doctors and their careers*, Policy Studies Institute, London, 1988.

18. Barrett, M. and Roberts, H., 'Why do women go to the doctor?' Paper given to the British Sociological Association, Manchester, 1976.

19. Lever, J., *PMT The Unrecogniqed Illness*, The New English Library/Times Mirror, London, 1980.

20. Sandler, M., *Personal Communication*, 1987.

21. MacIntyre, S., 'Communications between Pregnant Women and their Medical and Midwifery Attendants', *Midwives Chronicle and Nursing Times*, November 1983; 387–394.

22. Barrie, H., 'Back to Nature', *Faculty News*, 1984; No 4 (2): 1–2.

23. McManus, I. C. and Richards, P., 'Admissions to Medical School', *British Medical Journal*, 1986; 290:319–320.

24. *Minutes of the Meeting of London University Senate*, 16th March 1988.

25. Gow, D., 'Students' race to be monitored,' *Guardian*, 2nd July, 1988, p 3.

26. Bhate, S., 'Prejudice against Doctors and Students from Ethnic Minorities', *British Medical Journal* 1987; 294: 838.

27. Patel, S., 'The Imperfect Practices', *Guardian*, 18th Dec 1986, p. 14.

28. *Overseas Doctors' Experience and Expectations*, Commission For Racial Equality, London, 1987.

29. McNaught, A., *Race and Health Care In the United Kingdom*, Occasional paper No. 2, Health Education Council, 1985.

30. Shaunack, S. Colston, K. Patel SP. & Maxwell, D., 'Vitamin deficiency in adult British Hindu Asians,' *British Medical Journal*, 1985; 291: 1166–1168.

31. Black, J., 'Paediatrics among Ethnic Minorities', *British Medical Journal*, 1985; 290: 615–617.

32. Black, J., 'Paediatrics among Ethnic Minorities,' *British Medical Journal*, 1985; 290: 689–690.

33. Lakhani, S. R., Abraham, R. and Maxwell, J. D., 'Differences amongst Asian Patients', *British Medical Journal*, 1986; 293: 1169.

34. Burke, A., 'Racism and Psychological Disturbance Among West Indians in Britain,' *International Journal of Psychiatry*, 1984; 30:50–67.

35. Littlewood R. and Lipsedge M., 'Psychiatric Illness among British Afro-Caribbeans', *British Medical Journal*, 1988; 296: 950–951.

36. Lipsedge, M. and Littlewood, R., *In Recent Advances in Psychiatry*, Edited by Granville-Grossman, K., Churchill Livingstone, Edinburgh, 1979.

37. Bolton, P., 'Management of compulsory Admitted Patients to a High Security Unit,' *International Journal Of Psychiatry*, 1984; 30: 77–84.

38. Hemminki, E. and Heikkil, A., 'Factors Influencing Drug Prescribing: an Inquiry into Research Strategy,' *Drug Intelligence and Clinical Pharmacology*, 1976; 10.

39. Brown GM and Harris T., *The Social Origins of Depression*, Tavistock Publications, London, 1978.

40. Foy, A., Drinkwater, V., March, S. and Mearrick, P., 'Confusion after admission to hospital in elderly patients using benzodiazepines', *British Medical Journal*, 1986; 293: 1071.

41. Bloor, M. J., Venters G. A. and Samphier, M. L., 'Geographical Variation in the Incidence of Operations on the Tonsils and Adenoids,' *Journal of Laryngology and Otology*, 1978; 92: 791–801.

42. Adams, I. D., Chan, M., Clifford, P. C., Cooke, W. M. et al., 'Computer aided diagnosis of acute abdominal pain: a multicentre study', *British Medical Journal*, 1986; 293: 800–804.

43. *Report of a survey of medical education practices in United Kingdom Medical Schools*, General Medical Council, London, 1988.

44. *Recommendations on General Clinical Training*, General Medical Council, London, 1987.

45. *National Conference on the role of the doctor in New Zealand: Implications for Medical Education*, Summary report of a meeting held in Palmerston North, October 1985.

46. Collier Joe, 'Restricting Drugs', *Marxism Today*, April 1985, p 4–5.

47. Collier, Joe & Foster, John, 'Management of a restricted drugs policy in hospital: the first five years' experience,' *Lancet*, 1985; 1:331–333.

48. Davenas, E. Beauvais F, Amara, M. Oberbaum, M et al., 'Human basophil degranulation triggered by very dilute antiserum against IgE,' *Nature*, 1988; 333:816–818.

49. 'Herbal Medicines – Safe and Effective?', *Drug and Therapeutics Bulletin'*, 1986; 24:97–100.

50. Baker, S. and Thomas, P. S., 'Herbal Medicines Precipitating Massive Haemolysis', *Lancet*, 1987; 1:1039–1040.

51. *Annual Reports of the Medicines Commission and Section – 4 Committees for 1985*, page 37, published by the DHSS, July 1986.

52. *Which?*, Consumers' Association; London, October 1987.

Chapter 2: In the Pocket of the Industry

1 *Report of the Committee of Enquiry into the Relationship of the Pharmaceutical Industry with the National Health Service*, 1965–7, HMSO, London, 1967.

2 Data from the Office of Health Economics, 1987.

3. Collier, J. G., 'The Pharmaceutical Price Regulation Scheme: A Time for Change', *Lancet* 1985; 1:862–863.

4. Wilson, D., 'Freedom of information the loser in Section 2 reform,' *Guardian*, 1st July 1988: page 20.

5. *Scrip 1987*; No 1301: p 2.

6. Memo to Beecham Pharmaceuticals from Peter Woods, Mark Clark and David Morgan of Barclays de Zoete Wedd, 19 May 1987.

7 Nicholson, R., Research Investment – The key to Successful Science Based Industry, Upjohn Lecture. 21st October, 1986.

8. *New Scientist*, IPC Magazines Ltd, 3rd December 1987.

9. Medawar, C., *The Wrong Kind of Medicine*, published by Consumers' Association and Hodder and Stoughton; 1984.

10. 'Does Stanozolol Prevent Venous Ulceration?', *Drug and Therapeutics Bulletin 1985*; 23:91–92.

11. British National Formulary.

12. *New Focus on Pharmaceuticals*, Report by the National Economic Development Office, HMSO; 1986.

13. Radford, T., 'Vaccine prices will cost lives,' *Guardian* 11 March 1988; page 3.

14. *Scrip 1987*, No. 1196, p. 3.

15. Report of the Royal College of Physicians: The Relationship Between Physicians and the Pharmaceutical Industry,' *Journal of the Royal College of Physicians of London 1986*; 20:235–242.

16. de Bruxelles, S. and Wilson, B., 'Top Doctor Quits in Fees Row,' *Observer* 21st December 1986.

17. *Scrip 1987*; No 1196:3.

18. *Scrip 1988*; No 1301:8.

19. *Pharmaprojects 1987*; Volume 8. Published by V & O Publications Ltd, Richmond, Surrey.

20. *Scrip 1986*; No 1159:15.

21. Green David G., *Medicines In the Market Place*, Published by the Institute of Economic Affairs; London, 1987.

22. *New Focus on Pharmaceuticals*, HMSO; 1987.

23. Mann, R. D., *Orphan Diseases for orphan drugs*, edited by Scheinbertg, I. H. and Walshe, J. M., Manchester University Press 1986; 146–149.

24. Data Presented to the Clinical Section of the British Pharmacological Society, January 1988.

25. *Medicines Act*, Section 130, 2.

26. Orme, M., 'Aspirin all round?', *British Medical Journal*, 1988; 296:307–308.

27. Howie, J., *Ten years on from Swann*, The Association of Veterinarians in Industry, London 1981.

28. 'Clinical Trials of Antihistaminic Drugs in the Prevention and treatment of the Common Cold,' Report by a Special Committee of the Medical Research Council, *British Medical Journal*, 1950; 2:425–429.

29. Lock, S., *A Difficult Balance: Editorial Pier Review in Medicine*, published by the Nuffield Provincial Hospitals Trust; 1985.

30. Hampton J. R. and Julian D. G., 'Role of the Pharmaceutical Industry in Major Clinical Trials,' *Lancet* 1987; 2:1258–1259.

31. Lauritsen, K., Havelund, T., Laursen, L. S. and Rask-Madsen, 'Withholding Unfavourable Results in Drug Company Sponsored Clinical Trials,' *Lancet* 1987; 1:1091.

32. *Annual Reports of the Medicines Commission and Section-4 Committees for 1985*, published by the DHSS July 1986; page 1.

33. Hansard, *Written Answers* 26th Feb 1988: Column 364.

34. Ferriman, A., 'Exposed: Drug Firm's Hard Sell Line To Doctors,' *Observer* 9th June 1986; Page 3.

35. Erlichman, J., 'Company Tested Heart Drug Without DHSS Clearance,' *Guardian* 3 Nov, 1986, p 6.

36. Bland, J. M., Jones, D. R., Bennet, S., Cook, D. G. et al., 'Is the Clinical Trial Evidence about New Drugs Statistically Adequate?,' *British Journal of Clinical Pharmacology*, 1985; 19:155–160.

37. 'Tiaprofenic Acid (Surgam) – A Major Claim is Dropped,' *Drug and Therapeutics Bulletin*, 1983; 21:49–50.

38. *Prescription Event Monitoring News*, published by Innman, 1987.

39. Erlichman, J., 'The Bogus Drugs Testing at Heart of Sales Drive Aimed at GPs', *Guardian* Sept 10th 1986, page 3.

40. Bayer Company Internal Memo; 17th Nov 1983.

41. *Drug and Therapeutics Bulletin*, 1985; 25:1–3.

42. Collier, J. Drug trials – the search for safety. *The Times*. 13th May 1985, p. 10.

43. Thompson, I. E., French, K., Melia, K. M. et al., 'Research Ethics Committees in Scotland,' *British Medical Journal*, 1981; 282: 718–720.

44. Allen, P. A. and Waters, W. E., 'A Survey of Research Ethical Committees in Wessex in 1981', *Public Health*, London, 1982; 96:365–367.

45. 'British Medical Association Local Ethical Committees,' *British Medical Journal*, 1981; 282: 1010.

46. *Report of an Institute of Medical Ethics working group, Research Ethics Committees in Medical Research with Children: Ethics Law and Practice*, edited by Nicholson, R. H., published by Oxford University Press, 1986.

47. 'Research on healthy volunteers. A report of the Royal College of Physicians', *Journal of the Royal College of Physicians of London*, 1986; 20:243–257.

48. *Advice to health ministers on healthy volunteer studies*, DHSS, June 1987.

49. McFarlane A., 'The Downs and Ups of Infant Mortality,' *British Medical Journal*, 1988; 296:230–231.

50. Anon. 'Too Many H_2 Antagonists', *Lancet*, 1988; 1:28–29.

51. 'Rational Use of Vitamins,' *Drug and Therapeutics Bulletin*, 1984; 22:33–36.

52. Collier J. G. and New L., 'Illegibility of Drug Advertisements,' *Lancet* 1984; 1:341–342.

53. Collier J. G., 'Rules of Conduct and the Pharmaceutical Industry,' *Lancet*, 1984; 1:453.

54. Collier J. G., 'The Medicines Act and the ABPI Code,' *Lancet* 1984; 1:682–683.

55. Collier J. G. and Pilkington T. R. E., 'Human Insulin: a Misleading Advertisement,' *British Medical Journal*, 1984; 289:191.

56. *Today*, BBC Radio 4, Monday 4th May 1984.

57. Cox P., 'Rules of Conduct and the Pharmaceutical Industry,' *Lancet*, 1984; 1:517.

58. *Newsnight*, BBC2, September 12th 1984.

59. McKenna W. J., Rowlands E. and Krikler D. M., 'Amiodarone: The Experience of the Last Decade,' *British Medical Journal*, 1983; 287: 1654–1656.

60. Anon. 'Amiodarone – When and for Whom?,' *Lancet* 1983; 2:1123–1124.

61. Collier J., Herxheimer A., 'Roussel convicted of misleading promotion,' *Lancet* 1987; 1:113–114.

62. Good, C. S., 'MDU Support,' *Journal of the Medical Defence Union*, 1987; Summer Edition: page 22.
63. Collier, Joe & Herxheimer, Andrew, 'Medicines Act passes crucial test,' *Lancet*, 1988; 1:1349.

Chapter 3: Government: the Double Agent

1 *The National Health Service Act*, 1946.
2. *Health Services Management: Implementation of the NHS Management Inquiry Report*, DHSS, HC(84)13. 1984.
3. MacFarlane A., 'The Downs and Ups of Infant Mortality,' *British Medical Journal* 1988; 296:230–231.
4. *Social Trends 18*, HMSO; London 1988.
5. 'Financing and Delivering Health Care. A Comparative Analysis of OECD Countries,' *OECD Social Policy Studies*, No. 4. 1987.
6. Anon. "MP asks why fourth heart child died." *Guardian*, 27th February 1988, p. 3.
7. Spokesperson for the DHSS. April 1988.
8. Company donations to the Conservative party and other political associations,' *Labour Party Policy Directorate*, 1987; no 77.
9. Sainsbury, Lord (Chairman): *Report of the Committee of Enquiry into the Relationship of the Pharmaceutical Industry with the National Health Service*. London HMSO 1967.
10. *Current Problems*, Number 21, published by the Committee on Safety of Medicines, January 1988.
11. Collier, J. G., 'Licensing and Provision of Medicines in the United Kingdom,' *Lancet* 1985; 2:377–381.
12. Erlichman, J., 'Food Watchdog Denies Conflict of Interest,' *Guardian* July 20th 1987; page 4.
13. *Annual Reports For 1987 of the Medicines Commission and the Section 4 Committees*, HMSO 1988.
14. 'Rules Governing Medicaments in the European Community,' *Council Directive* 20th May, 1975: 75/318/EEC.
15. *DataSheetforAllpyral*,PublishedbyDohme/Hollister-Stier;1986.
16. Anon., 'Mianserin 10 Years On,' *Drug and Therapeutics Bulletin*, 1988; 26; 17–18.
17. *British National Formulary*, 1988; 15:100–101.
18. Anon., 'Doubts About Dipyradamole as an Antithrombotic Drug,' *Drug and Therapeutics Bulletin*, 1984; 22:25–28.
19. Anon., 'Does Stanozolol prevent venous ulceration?', *Drug and Therapeutics Bulletin*, 1985; 23:91–92.

REFERENCES

20. Anon., 'Fluvoxamine (Faverin): Another Antidepressive Drug,' *Drug and Therapeutics Bulletin*, 1988; 26;11–12.

21. Anon., 'Domperidone: an alternative to metaclopizmide', *Drug and Therapeutics Bulletin*, 1988. 26: 58–59.

22. Anon., *Drug and Therapeutics Bulletin*, 1988. In press.

23. Anon., 'Buspirone – A Radical Advance in the Treatment of Anxiety?', *Lancet*, 1988; 1:804–806.

24. Anon., 'Co-Trimoxazole, or just Trimethoprim?', *Drug and Therapeutics Bulletin*, 1986; 24:17–19.

25. Hodsman, G. P. and Robertson, J. I. S., 'Captopril: Five Years On.', *British Medical Journal*, 1983; 287:851–852.

26. Ballantyne, A., 'Patients get overdose of radiation,' *Guardian* Sat 24 July 1988, page 1.

27. Nicholson, A. N., 'Hypnotics: Their place in therapeutics,' *Drugs* 1986; 31:164–176.

28. Faich, G. A., Morrison, J., Dutra, E. V., Hare, D. B. and Rheinstein, P. H., 'Reassurance about generic drugs,' *New England Journal of Medicine*, 1987; 316:1473–1475.

29. Griffin, J. P. and Weber, J. C. P., 'Voluntary Systems of Adverse Reaction Reporting-Parts 1 and 2', *Adverse Drug Reactions and Accidental Poisoning Review*, 1985; 4:213–230 and 1986; 1:23–55.

30. Anon., 'Phenylbutazone and Oxyphenbutazone – A Time to Call A Halt', *Drug and Therapeutics Bulletin*, 1984; 22; 5–6.

31. McBride W. G., 'Thalidomide and congenital abnormalities,' *Lancet*, 1961; 2:1358.

32. Speirs, C. J., Griffin, J. P., Weber, J. C. P., Glen-Bott, M., Twomey, C. S., 'Demography of the UK Adverse Reactions Register of Spontaneous Reports,' *Health Trends*, 1984; 16:49–52.

33. *Current Problems* March 1987, No 19. Issued by the Committee on Safety of Medicines.

34. Erlichman, J., 'Computers to win over the doctors'. *Guardian*, 9th September, 1987: page 33.

35. *Medicines Act Information Leaflet*, 1987; number 19, appendix 3.

36. Evans N. J. B. and Cunliffe P. W., *Study of Control of Medicines*, HMSO; London, 1987.

37. Anon., 'When to try alternate-day corticosteroid therapy,' *Drug and Therapeutics Bulletin*, 1976; 14:49–51.

38. Bain, R., 'Variations in Drug Quality,' *The Proprietary Articles Trade Association Official Reference Book*, 1987; pp. 33–35.

39. Anon., 'Inactive ingredients in medicines,' *Lancet*, 1988; 1:1143–1144.

163

40. Wells, F., 'Disclosure of inactive ingredients,' *Lancet*, 1988; 1:1339.

41. 'CSM Update,' *British Medical Journal*, 1988; 296:1319.

42. Ferriman, A., 'Pep-up drug deaths,' *Observer*, 5 June 1988, page 1.

43. DHSS Press release 88/191, 1988.

44. *Annual Reports of the Medicines Commission and Section-4 Committees for 1985*, Published by the DHSS; July 1986.

45. Timmins N., 'Alarm at Ruling on Drug Licences', *Independent* 1987; 30th December.

46. Brahams, D., 'Drug Licensing Authority's Use of Originator's Confidential Data,' *Lancet*, 1988; 2:116.

47. Fitzgerald, G. A., 'Drug Therapy: Dipyradomole,' *New England Journal Of Medicine*, 1987; 316: 1247–1250.

48. 'CSM Update; Non-steroid Anti-inflammatory Drugs and Serious Gastrointestinal Adverse Reactions,' *British Medical Journal*, 1986; 292:614.

49. Medawar Charles, 'Data Sheets: A consumer Perspective,' *Lancet*, 1988; 1: 777–8.

50. Anon., 'Transdermal glyceryl trinitrate patches (Transiderm-nitro)', *Drug and Therapeutics Bulletin*, 1986; 24:5–6.

51. Anon., 'Nitrates: the problem of tolerance,' *Drug and Therapeutics Bulletin*, 1988; 26:57–59.

52. *Hansard*, 1985; 82: Column 561–562.

53. 'Private Question 3481,' *Hansard* 1986–87; 113: Column 75.

54. Dobson, F. and MacGarvin, M., *Cervical Cancer Screening: What's Going On?*, a report Prepared for Frank Dobson MP, March 1985.

55. Anon., 'Cervical Screening: A Promise Unfulfilled,' *Lancet* 1987; 1:877.

56. Elwood J. M., Cotton, R. E., Johnson, J., Jones G. M. et al., 'Are Patients with abnormal smears adequately managed?', *British Medical Journal*, 1984; 289; 891–894.

57. Veitch A., 'Specialists cast doubt on smear test deadline,' *Guardian*, 1987, December 8th: page 4.

58. Veitch A., 'Health Authorities unable to meet cancer screening deadline,' *Guardian*, 28th March, 1988; page 20.

59. Anon., 'The Forrest report', *Lancet*, 1987; 1:575.

60. DHSS Press Release 25th Feb. 1987, 87/78.

61. Veitch A., 'Fowler Puts £20m into Aids and Cancer Fight,' *Guardian*, 26 February 1987; p. 7.

62. *The Health Divide*, Published by the Health Education Council, March 1987.

63. *Heart Beat Wales*, Report Number 7: Pulse of Wales, published by Heart Beat Wales; 1987.
64. Registrar General's Decennial Supplement Life Tables, 1981.
65. Gardner M. and Donnan S., 'Life Expectancy: Variations among regional Health Authorities,' *Population Trends*, Number 10, HMSO, 1978.
66. Townsend, P. and Davidson, N., *Inequalities in Health; The Black Report*, published by Penguin Books Ltd, 1982.
67. *The Health Divide*, published by the Health Education Council, March 1987.
68. *Inequalities in Health*, Report of the Working Group on Inequalities in Health chaired by Sir Douglas Black, published by DHSS; 1980.
69. *Comparative Mortality From Drugs Of Addiction by the BMA and Action on Alcohol Abuse Publication*, published by BMA; 1987.
70. Anon., 'A Mockery of Health Promotion,' *Lancet*, 1987; 1:489.
71. *Action on Smoking at Work*, Health Education Council; 1985.

Chapter 4: Patient, Heal Thyself

1. Dunnell K., Cartwright A., *Medicine Takers, Hoarders and Prescribers*, Routledge and Kegan Paul; London, 1972.
2. Collier J. G. & Anderson H. R., Unpublished Data.
3. *General Household Survey*, HMSO; London, 1985.
4. *Social Trends Number 18*, HMSO; London, 1988.
5. Tuckett D., Boulton, M., Olson C. and Williams, A., *Meetings between Experts*, Tavistock Publications; 1985.
6. Valanis B., Rumpler C., *Cancer Nursing*, 1985; 8:167–175.
7. McManus, I., *British Medical Journal*, 1988, in press.
8. Jones, L. Leneman, L. & Maclean U., *Consumer feedback for the NHS*, published by King Edward's Hospital Fund for London, 1987.
9. Dyer C., 'Master of the Rolls says doctors must exxplain if things go wrong,' *Guardian* 25 March 1988; Page 4.
10. Brahams D., 'Doctor's Duty to Answer Patients' Inquiries,' *Lancet*, 1987; 1:932.
11. *Medicines (leaflets) Regulations*, 1977.
12. Anon., 'Reporting Adverse Reactions: the Black Triangle and the Patient, *Drug and Therapeutics Bulletin*, 1983; 21:93–94.
13. Herxheimer A., 'Detecting Adverse Reactions to Medicines,' *Self Health*, 1988; Issue 18:15–16.
14. Anon, 'Disease Education By the BBC, *British Medical Journal*, 1958; 1:388–389.
15. Fletcher, C. M., *Personal Communication*, 1987.

Index